Management of Labor and Delivery

Editor

AARON B. CAUGHEY

OBSTETRICS AND GYNECOLOGY CLINICS OF NORTH AMERICA

www.obgyn.theclinics.com

Consulting Editor
WILLIAM F. RAYBURN

December 2017 • Volume 44 • Number 4

ELSEVIER

1600 John F. Kennedy Boulevard ● Suite 1800 ● Philadelphia, Pennsylvania, 19103-2899

http://www.theclinics.com

OBSTETRICS AND GYNECOLOGY CLINICS OF NORTH AMERICA Volume 44, Number 4
December 2017 ISSN 0889-8545, ISBN-13: 978-0-323-55286-8

Editor: Kerry Holland
Developmental Editor: Kristen Helm

Obstetrics and Gynecology Clinics (ISSN 0889-8545) is published quarterly by Elsevier Inc., 360 Park Avenue South, New York, NY 10010-1710. Months of issue are March, June, September, and December. Periodicals postage paid at New York, NY, and additional mailing offices. Subscription price per year is $301.00 (US individuals), $627.00 (US institutions), $100.00 (US students), $377.00 (Canadian individuals), $792.00 (Canadian institutions), $225.00 (Canadian students), $459.00 (international individuals), $792.00 (international institutions), and $225.00 (international students). To receive student/resident rate, orders must be accompanied by name of affiliated institution, date of term, and the signature of program/residency coordinator on institution letterhead. Orders will be billed at individual rate until proof of status is received. Foreign air speed delivery is included in all Clinics subscription prices. All prices are subject to change without notice. POSTMASTER: Send address changes to Obstetrics and Gynecology Clinics, Elsevier Health Sciences Division, Subscription Customer Service, 3251 Riverport Lane, Maryland Heights, MO 63043. **Customer Service: Telephone: 1-800-654-2452 (U.S. and Canada); 314-447-8871 (outside U.S. and Canada). Fax: 314-447-8029. E-mail: journalscustomerservice-usa@elsevier.com (for print support); journalsonlinesupport-usa@elsevier.com (for online support).**

Reprints. For copies of 100 or more of articles in this publication, please contact the Commercial Reprints Department, Elsevier Inc., 360 Park Avenue South, New York, New York 10010-1710. Tel.: 212-633-3874; Fax: 212-633-3820; E-mail: reprints@elsevier.com.

Obstetrics and Gynecology Clinics of North America is also published in Spanish by McGraw-Hill Interamericana Editores S.A., P.O. Box 5-237, 06500, Mexico; in Portuguese by Reichmann and Affonso Editores, Rio de Janeiro, Brazil; and in Greek by Paschalidis Medical Publications, Athens, Greece.

Obstetrics and Gynecology Clinics of North America is covered in MEDLINE/PubMed (Index Medicus), Excerpta Medica, Current Concepts/Clinical Medicine, Science Citation Index, BIOSIS, CINAHL, and ISI/BIOMED.

Contributors

CONSULTING EDITOR

WILLIAM F. RAYBURN, MD, MBA
Associate Dean, Continuing Medical Education and Professional Development, Distinguished Professor and Emeritus Chair, Obstetrics and Gynecology, University of New Mexico School of Medicine, Albuquerque, New Mexico

EDITOR

AARON B. CAUGHEY, MD, PhD
Professor and Chair, Department of Obstetrics and Gynecology, Oregon Health & Science University, Portland, Oregon

AUTHORS

ALLISON J. ALLEN, MD
Maternal-Fetal Medicine Fellow, Department of Obstetrics and Gynecology, Oregon Health & Science University, Portland, Oregon

ALISON G. CAHILL, MD, MSCI
Associate Professor, Department of Obstetrics and Gynecology, Chief, Division of Maternal-Fetal Medicine, Washington University School of Medicine in St. Louis, St Louis, Missouri

AARON B. CAUGHEY, MD, PhD
Professor and Chair, Department of Obstetrics and Gynecology, Oregon Health & Science University, Portland, Oregon

YVONNE W. CHENG, MD, PhD
Medical Director, Division of Maternal-Fetal Medicine, Department of Obstetrics and Gynecology, Sutter Health, California Pacific Medical Center, San Francisco, California; Department of Surgery, University of California, Davis, Davis, California

NATHAN S. FOX, MD
Maternal-Fetal Medicine Associates, PLLC, Department of Obstetrics, Gynecology, and Reproductive Science, Icahn School of Medicine at Mount Sinai, New York, New York

ANNESSA KERNBERG, MD
Department of Obstetrics and Gynecology, Oregon Health & Science University, Portland, Oregon

BETH LEOPOLD, MD
Resident, Department of Obstetrics and Gynecology, Christiana Care Health System, Newark, Delaware

SARAH E. LITTLE, MD, MPH
Assistant Professor, Division of Maternal-Fetal Medicine, Brigham and Women's Hospital, Harvard Medical School, Boston, Massachusetts

STEPHANIE MELKA, MD
Maternal-Fetal Medicine Associates, PLLC, Department of Obstetrics, Gynecology, and Reproductive Science, Icahn School of Medicine at Mount Sinai, New York, New York

JAMES MILLER, MD
Maternal-Fetal Medicine Associates, PLLC, Department of Obstetrics, Gynecology, and Reproductive Science, Icahn School of Medicine at Mount Sinai, New York, New York

CHRISTINA A. PENFIELD, MD, MPH
Clinical Instructor and Maternal-Fetal Medicine Fellow, Department of Obstetrics and Gynecology, School of Medicine, University of California, Irvine, Orange, California

RACHEL A. PILLIOD, MD
Clinical Fellow, Department of Obstetrics and Gynecology, Division of Maternal-Fetal Medicine, Oregon Health & Science University, Portland, Oregon

NANDINI RAGHURAMAN, MD, MS
Maternal-Fetal Medicine Fellow, Department of Obstetrics and Gynecology, Division of Maternal-Fetal Medicine, Washington University School of Medicine in St. Louis, St Louis, Missouri

JANINE S. RHOADES, MD
Department of Obstetrics and Gynecology, Washington University School of Medicine in St. Louis, St Louis, Missouri

BETHANY SABOL, MD
Department of Obstetrics and Gynecology, Oregon Health & Science University, Portland, Oregon

JAMES SARGENT, MD
Clinical Fellow in Maternal-Fetal Medicine, Department of Obstetrics and Gynecology, Oregon Health & Science University, Portland, Oregon

ANTHONY SCISCIONE, DO
Director of Maternal-Fetal Medicine and the OB/Gyn Residency Program, Department of Obstetrics and Gynecology, Christiana Care Health System, Newark, Delaware

DEBORAH A. WING, MD, MBA
Professor, Department of Obstetrics and Gynecology, School of Medicine, University of California, Irvine, Orange, California

Contents

This article provides an overview of the approaches that might be used to safely reduce the cesarean rate. Although cesarean delivery may be a safe alternative to vaginal delivery, its use in 1 in 3 women giving birth is likely too high. The downstream impact of cesarean delivery on future pregnancies is likely not well considered when the first cesarean is being performed. Through quality improvement, environmental changes will allow clinicians to adopt the range of practices described. However, without such environmental changes, clinicians may not be able to change their own practice patterns given environments in which they practice.

Modern data have redefined the normal first stage of labor. Key differences include that the latent phase of labor is much slower than was previously thought and the transition from latent to active labor does not occur until about 6 cm of cervical dilatation, regardless of parity or whether labor was spontaneous or induced. Providers should have a low threshold to use one of the safe and effective interventions to manage abnormal progression in the first stage of labor, including oxytocin, internal tocodynamometry, and amniotomy.

The American College of Obstetricians and Gynecologists (ACOG) Practice Bulletin No. 49 on Dystocia and Augmentation of Labor defines a prolonged second stage as more than 2 hours without or 3 hours with epidural analgesia in nulliparous women, and 1 hour without or 2 hours with epidural in multiparous women. This definition diagnoses 10% to 14% of nulliparous and 3% to 3.5% of multiparous women as having a prolonged second stage. Although current labor norms remained largely based on data established by Friedman in the 1950s, modern obstetric population and practice have evolved with time.

Electronic fetal monitoring (EFM) is widely used to assess fetal status in labor. Use of intrapartum continuous EFM is associated with a lower risk of neonatal seizures but a higher risk of cesarean or operative delivery. Category II fetal heart tracings are indeterminate in their ability to predict fetal acidemia. Certain patterns of decelerations and variability within this category may be predictive of neonatal morbidity. Adjunct tests of fetal well-being can be used during labor to further triage patients. Intrauterine resuscitation techniques should target the suspected etiology of intrapartum fetal hypoxia. Clinical factors play a role in the interpretation of EFM.

The laborist movement was introduced as a means to improve the quality of care patients receive in the labor suite and decrease physician burnout and malpractice claims. This model of care has rapidly expanded, and there is evidence of its potential role in improving labor outcomes. This article outlines the different models of laborist care, reviews the evidence for its potential impact on labor outcomes, and discusses the economic impact the employment of laborists can have.

Fetal malpresentation and fetal malposition are frequently interchanged; however, fetal malpresentation refers to a fetus with a fetal part other than the head engaging the maternal pelvis. Fetal malposition in labor includes occiput posterior and occiput transverse positions. Both fetal malposition and malpresentation are associated with significant maternal and neonatal morbidity, which have significant impact on patients and providers. Accurate diagnosis of both conditions is necessary for appropriate management. In this article, terminology, incidence, diagnosis, and management are discussed.

Obstetricians who care for twin pregnancies should be aware of the challenges that may arise during the labor and delivery. With recognition of these issues and proper training, providers should be able to help women with twin pregnancies achieve a safe delivery for them and their babies. With the use of breech extraction of the second twin and active management of the second stage of labor, women with twin pregnancies can also achieve a high vaginal delivery rate of both twins.

The cesarean delivery rate has plateaued at 32%; concurrently, after peaking in the mid-1990s, trial of labor after cesarean (TOLAC) rates have declined. Less than 25% of women with a prior cesarean delivery attempt a future TOLAC. This decreasing trend in TOLAC is caused by inadequate resource availability, malpractice concerns, and lack of knowledge in patients and providers regarding the perceived risks and benefits. This article outlines the factors influencing recent vaginal birth after cesarean trends in addition to reviewing the maternal and neonatal outcomes associated with TOLAC, specifically in high-risk populations.

There has been an emphasis on redesigning our health care system to eliminate medical errors and create a culture of safety. The American College of Obstetrics and Gynecologists defines a culture of safety as an environment in which all care providers are empowered to identify errors, near misses, risky behaviors, and broader systems issues while engaging in active collaboration to improve and resolve processes and system failures. This article reviews key components that promote a culture of safety and help to implement safer, more effective, evidence-based quality care on labor and delivery units.

OBSTETRICS AND GYNECOLOGY CLINICS

Foreword

Addressing Common Management Dilemmas in Labor and Delivery

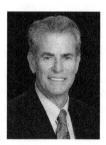

William F. Rayburn, MD, MBA
Consulting Editor

This issue of the *Obstetrics and Gynecology Clinics of North America* deals with key management decisions undertaken regularly in the Labor and Delivery Unit. Ably edited by Aaron Caughey, MD, the issue highlights controversies pertaining to induction of labor, progression during the first and second stages, fetal monitoring interpretation, reducing cesarean delivery rates, and enhancing quality care and patient safety.

Management during labor and delivery requires two views: (1) acceptance of a normal physiologic process that most women experience, and (2) anticipation of complications, often occurring unexpectedly and quickly. Labor onset represents the culmination of a series of biochemical changes in the cervix and uterus. Preterm labor, dystocia, and postterm pregnancy may result when labor is abnormal.

Induction of labor affects one in every four pregnancies, although the incidence varies between practices. Topics covered by the authors pertain to the role of outpatient preinduction cervical ripening, best techniques for labor induction, and impact of elective induction of labor. Oxytocin for inducing or augmenting labor is common, affecting half or more of all pregnancies undergoing a trial of labor. Use of oxytocin for augmentation and active labor is well reviewed in this issue.

Many abnormalities may interfere with the orderly progression of fetal descent and spontaneous vaginal delivery. Soon after admission, a rational plan for monitoring labor can be established based on past pregnancies and current needs of the fetus and mother. Because there are marked variations in labor lengths, precise statements are unwise as to its anticipated duration.

Electronic measurement of uterine activity permits generalities about certain contraction patterns and labor outcome. Uterine muscle efficiency to effect delivery varies greatly. Abnormal progress during the first and second stages of labor is defined

Obstet Gynecol Clin N Am 44 (2017) xi–xii
https://doi.org/10.1016/j.ogc.2017.09.002
0889-8545/17/© 2017 Published by Elsevier Inc.

obgyn.theclinics.com

in this issue along with principles of management. Slow progress arises from a single or combination of several factors: insufficiently strong or coordinated uterine contractions; fetal malpresentations or malpositioning; abnormalities of the maternal pelvis creating a contracted pelvis; soft tissue restrictions in the lower reproductive tract; and inadequate maternal pushing during the second stage. These abnormalities are addressed categorically in this issue.

Electronic fetal monitoring was introduced into practice 50 years ago. The continuously recorded fetal heart rate pattern is potentially diagnostic in assessing pathophysiologic events. Accurate information provided by this monitoring remains a matter of debate, however, despite most American women now being monitored electronically during labor. The authors focus on category II tracings, which include those characterized as being neither normal (category I) nor abnormal (category III). A systematic analysis of the baseline rate, baseline variability, accelerations, and periodic or episodic decelerations is described.

Also, over the past 50 years, the cesarean delivery rate in the United States rose from 5% to 33%. This rate declined temporarily, mostly from a significant increase of vaginal births after cesarean (VBAC), and to a closely mirrored decrease in primary cesareans. Reasons for this high cesarean rate relate to the following conditions: common performance of a repeat cesarean; use of electronic monitoring with a resultant higher suspicion of "fetal distress"; breech-presenting fetus delivered by cesarean; operative vaginal deliveries being performed less; labor induction being more common, especially among nulliparas; maternal obesity being observed frequently; more cesareans being performed for women with preeclampsia; lower VBAC rates; elective cesarean deliveries to avoid pelvic floor injury or reduce fetal risk or upon maternal request; and fear of litigation. Many of these conditions are covered in this issue.

The authors emphasize the growing need for quality improvement and patient safety on labor and delivery and how it may be measured for a variety of conditions. This trend was accompanied by the evolution of the laborist movement in the United States. Much of this has arisen to provide care that is more standard and accessible. The American College of Obstetricians and Gynecologists and the American Academy of Pediatrics continue to collaborate in the development of guidelines for optimal care in labor and delivery. These efforts are intended to improve interdisciplinary communication, increase team-based effort with clarified expectations, and increase engagement in decision-making with the patient and family. While these guidelines apply to all pregnancies, they are especially relevant to twin pregnancies as covered in this issue.

Management strategies addressed here should be helpful to the obstetrician during labor and delivery. Dr Caughey did well in selecting an accomplished group of authors with proven clinical and research experience in their field. Evidence-based approaches imparted in this collection are greatly appreciated for immediate use and future direction.

William F. Rayburn, MD, MBA
Continuing Medical Education &
Professional Development
MSC 10 5580, 1 University of New Mexico
Albuquerque, NM 87131-0001, USA

E-mail address:
WRayburn@salud.unm.edu

Preface

Evidence-Based Management of Labor and Delivery: What Do We Still Need to Know?

 CrossMark

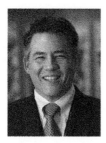

Aaron B. Caughey, MD, PhD
Editor

In the United States, there are four million births each year, and the large majority of them occur in hospitals on labor and delivery units.[1] These specialized locations are so specific that really only pregnant women can use this space, and an enormous amount of resources is dedicated to the care of pregnant women going through the birth process. Why would we have women who are experiencing a normal physiologic event in the majority of cases, do so in the hospital? Predominantly this is because of the small, but specific, inherent risk that accompanies childbirth, both to mothers and to babies. Over the twentieth century, a number of interventions were developed and refined to reduce the morbidity and mortality for mothers and babies, including blood banking, antibiotics, and more specifically, fetal heart rate monitoring and operative obstetrics, notably the cesarean delivery.

At this point in the twenty-first century, there are more than 1.2 million cesarean deliveries each year in the United States.[2] While a cesarean rate above 15% to 20% appears to be associated with lower maternal and neonatal mortality, a benefit by increasing the cesarean rate up to the current 32% in the United States has not been demonstrated.[3] The divide between these two thresholds has been a focus for the past decade. One of the drivers identified to safely reduce the primary cesarean rate is the use of more evidence-based labor and delivery management.[4]

The collection of articles in this issue of *Obstetrics and Gynecology Clinics of North America* deals with just that, the evidence-based management of labor and delivery. While many are framed with the focus on mode of delivery and the potential for reducing the cesarean rate, the intent is to provide the most up-to-date evidence to guide practice, research, and contemplation of obstetric management. The articles include more general management of labor and fetal heart rate monitoring as well as

Obstet Gynecol Clin N Am 44 (2017) xiii–xiv
https://doi.org/10.1016/j.ogc.2017.09.001
0889-8545/17/© 2017 Published by Elsevier Inc.

more specific articles on twins, malposition, and malpresentation. There are also pieces on laborist models and quality improvement on labor and delivery. Throughout them all, I think you will see that while there has been an increasing amount of evidence produced over the past several decades, there is a great need for much more evidence to be accumulated on specifics of labor and delivery care.

So, if you have a passion for labor and delivery as I do, I hope you enjoy this collection of pieces and will be inspired after reading to identify some holes in the existing research and start a research project to address a question or begin a quality improvement project to improve outcomes. Enjoy, and I hope to see you on L&D!

Aaron B. Caughey, MD, PhD
Department of Obstetrics and Gynecology
Oregon Health & Science University
3181 SW Sam Jackson Park Road
Portland, OR 97239, USA

E-mail address:
caughey@ohsu.edu

REFERENCES

1. MacDorman MF, Matthews TJ, Declercq E. Trends in out-of-hospital births in the United States, 1990-2012. NCHS Data Brief 2014;(144):1–8.
2. Martin JA, Hamilton BE, Osterman MJ, et al. Births: final data for 2015. Natl Vital Stat Rep 2017;66(1):1.
3. Molina G, Weiser TG, Lipsitz SR, et al. Relationship between cesarean delivery rate and maternal and neonatal mortality. JAMA 2015;314(21):2263–70.
4. American College of Obstetricians and Gynecologists (College); Society for Maternal-Fetal Medicine, Caughey AB, Cahill AG, Guise JM, et al. Safe prevention of the primary cesarean delivery. Am J Obstet Gynecol 2014;210(3):179–93.

Evidence-Based Labor and Delivery Management

Can We Safely Reduce the Cesarean Rate?

Aaron B. Caughey, MD, PhD

KEYWORDS

- Evidence-based • Labor • Delivery • Management • Safety • Cesarean rate

KEY POINTS

- Although cesarean delivery may be an increasingly safe alternative to vaginal delivery, its use in 1 in 3 women giving birth is likely too high.
- Furthermore, the downstream impact of cesarean delivery on future pregnancies is likely not well-considered when the first cesarean is being performed.
- There are a range of practices that have become standard that should be carefully questioned and replaced by standardized, evidence-based practices to decrease the rate of cesarean deliveries safely.
- Through quality improvement efforts such as perinatal quality collaboratives, the environmental changes will allow clinicians to adopt the range of practices described.
- Without environmental changes, clinicians may not be able to change practice patterns that have been encouraged by the given environments in which they practice.

INTRODUCTION

More than 100 years ago, the normal physiologic process of birth began to be moved into hospitals. Although those initial moves were likely not specifically designed to improve pregnancy outcomes, it has led to dramatic reductions in both the maternal and neonatal mortality rates.[1,2] It also provided the opportunity to better understand the birth process through epidemiologic study and clinical trials that can examine the impact of interventions. In one of the earliest cohort studies, Dr Emmanuel Friedman prospectively studied the labor and delivery process and reported out labor norms.[3] Unfortunately, instead of an increasing number of studies, these norms were used to establish specific labor guidelines that have been shown to increase interventions without clear evidence of benefit. One of the biggest impacts of having birth in a hospital in combination with specific labor guidelines has been the increasing increase in cesarean deliveries.

Department of Obstetrics and Gynecology, Oregon Health & Science University, 3181 Southwest Sam Jackson Road, Mail Code: L-466, Portland, OR 97239, USA
E-mail address: caughey@ohsu.edu

Obstet Gynecol Clin N Am 44 (2017) 523–533
http://dx.doi.org/10.1016/j.ogc.2017.08.008   **obgyn.theclinics.com**
0889-8545/17/© 2017 Elsevier Inc. All rights reserved.

In 2015, the cesarean rate in the United States was 32.0%, meaning that more than 1.2 million women delivered via cesarean.[4] Although this rate remains high, there has been a modest reduction in the rate of cesarean births, decreasing from 32.9% to 32.0%. This nearly 1% reduction means that there are 40,000 fewer cesarean deliveries each year. Unfortunately, previously, from 1996 to 2009, the cesarean rate increased from 20.7% to 32.9%, a more than 50% increase, which was nearly 500,000 more cesarean deliveries each year.[5] This increase occurred despite guidance from *Healthy People 2010* and *Healthy People 2020* that set the primary cesarean rate at 15% and the primary cesarean rate in term, nulliparous women at 23.9%.[6] Furthermore, it does not seem that there is any benefit to a cesarean delivery above 20%. In a study of 179 countries around the globe, researchers found that although both maternal and neonatal mortality rates were reduced as cesarean rates increased to 19%, from 20% and up, there was no further reduction of either maternal or neonatal mortality.[2]

In addition to the statistics regarding the increase in cesarean deliveries, it is compelling to note the wide variation in cesarean delivery rates between institutions.[7] The rate varies between institutions, even when controlling for characteristics that would account for indicated cesarean deliveries.[8] Although such variation may depend on additional factors that differ between institutions, the variation seems to be too great to be based on consistent, evidence-based care at all institutions. Thus, there is a need to develop evidence-based care and disseminate practice guidelines to ensure that all women are managed in a fashion that gives them the best hope for a good outcome. Our profession needs to more rapidly develop and study approaches to manage labor and delivery and reduce both maternal and neonatal morbidity and mortality, but at the same time safely reduce the use of cesarean deliveries.

This article provides an overview considering what approaches might be used to safely reduce the cesarean rate. These concepts are simply meant to touch on a number of labor and delivery management areas. Most of these are discussed in much greater depth by the articles included in this issue of *Obstetrics and Gynecology Clinics of North America*. Specifically, the papers delve into the management of the first and second stages of labor, including induction of labor, fetal heart rate monitoring, the management of multiple gestations, breech presentations, malposition, women with prior cesarean deliveries, laborist models, and quality improvement measures on labor and delivery.

WHY IS THE CESAREAN RATE INCREASING?

One possible reason for the increase in the cesarean delivery rate may be that there has simply been an increase in the need for cesarean deliveries. The most common indication for a primary cesarean is cephalopelvic disproportion or arrest of progress in labor. Although it is unlikely that maternal pelvis size has changed over the past 3 decades, it is possible that birthweight has increased. In fact, there is evidence that there have been increases in the rate of macrosomia over the past 2 decades.[9] Another 2 issues that contribute to increasing rates of cesarean delivery, possibly through the mechanism of birthweight, are maternal obesity and gestational weight gain.[10,11] Without question, the proportion of obese women has increased over the past decade[12] and the even higher weight classes, such as "super obesity," are associated with even higher rates of cesarean deliveries.[13] Additionally, increased gestational weight gain has been associated with cesarean delivery and is commonly above standard guidelines.[14]

Another reason for increasing cesarean rates may be an increase in elective cesarean delivery, also know as cesarean delivery by maternal request (CDMR). Because CDMR is not listed among *International Classification of Disease,* 9th edition, codes, it is unclear what proportion of cesarean deliveries are due to CDMR. However, 1 recent study estimated the proportion to be as high as 4% of the cesarean deliveries performed in the United States.[15] Interestingly, CDMR is more common in several other countries, including Brazil, Taiwan, and Chile. In Chile, in a study that compared women receiving private care who had a cesarean rate of greater than 40% with women receiving public care, who had a cesarean rate of less than 20%, 8% of the women receiving private care and 11% of the women receiving public care stated a preference toward cesarean delivery with the vast majority preferring to deliver vaginally.[16] Thus, even in this setting, it is unclear that maternal preferences are driving the increase in the cesarean delivery rate. The topic of CDMR led to an National Institutes of Health State-of-the-Science conference in 2006. The statement from this meeting concluded that future research was necessary to examine both the, "current extent of CDMR and attitudes about it."[17] More recently, a study in the United States found that the vast majority of women would prefer to deliver vaginally, all else being equal.[18]

So, although some maternal demographics have changed and maternal preferences may account for a small proportion of cesarean deliveries, it seems that much of the increase in cesarean rates may be due to cultural pressures and norms. Some of these pressures are due to the medicolegal environment that obstetric clinicians face. In 1 study, surveyed physicians reported that they were more likely to perform a cesarean delivery in a number of scenarios if they had been sued recently or if they thought about being sued frequently.[19] In another study, the amount of tort reform was associated with cesarean deliveries, in particular, those states that had caps on noneconomic damages in lawsuits had lower overall cesarean rates and higher vaginal birth after cesarean (VBAC) rates.[20]

HOW DOES CESAREAN DELIVERY AFFECT PREGNANCY OUTCOMES?

With respect to the effect of cesarean delivery on maternal and neonatal outcomes, much is known. Generally, there are both positive and negative effects related to cesarean delivery on both the mother and her baby.[21] With respect to the mother, cesarean delivery has been associated with higher rates of maternal hemorrhage, infection, and even death.[22] However, a cesarean delivery is protective against perineal lacerations.[23] In turn, there is some evidence to suggest that vaginal delivery may be associated with pelvic organ prolapse and both fecal and urinary incontinence. Importantly, there are risks from a cesarean delivery on maternal outcomes in future pregnancies, such as the risk of a trial of labor after a cesarean delivery.[24] In particular, the risk of abnormal placentation that can lead to the need for a preterm delivery and/or cesarean hysterectomy, and can be complicated by severe maternal hemorrhage, should receive significant attention when considering the risks of a cesarean delivery.[25,26]

Regarding neonatal outcomes, cesarean delivery is associated with lower rates of intrapartum hypoxic injury and neonatal mortality.[27] Additionally, with vaginal delivery there is always a risk of shoulder dystocia and permanent brachial plexus injury. Alternatively, neonates delivered via cesarean seem to experience higher rates of transient tachypnea of the newborn and possibly primary pulmonary hypertension.[11] Similar to the mother, neonates in future pregnancies after a prior cesarean delivery are at increased risk. There seems to be an increased risk of stillbirth[28] and, in pregnancies that undergo a trial of labor after cesarean (TOLAC), uterine rupture carries a risk to the neonate. Additionally, pregnancies may need to be delivered before term if complicated by an abnormal placentation.

WHAT ARE THE POTENTIAL APPROACHES TO SAFELY REDUCING CESAREAN DELIVERIES?

Although there may be components of the increase in cesarean deliveries that are due to changing demographics of the population, it seems that much of the increase is due to economic and medicolegal pressures on obstetric providers that have led to culture changes on labor and delivery. As noted, the increase in cesarean deliveries from 1996 to 2009 pushed the overall cesarean rate in the United States well above the 15% to 20% threshold for benefit that has been identified and recommended. In addition to no improvements in maternal or neonatal mortality, there are potential morbidities from cesarean delivery, including higher risks of maternal hemorrhage and infection.[22] Additionally, there are risks from a cesarean delivery on outcomes in future pregnancies. There are the risks of a TOLAC,[24] of course, but receiving increased interest is the risk of abnormal placentation that can lead to the need for a preterm delivery and/or cesarean hysterectomy, and can be complicated by severe maternal hemorrhage.[25,26]

Thus, the cesarean rate is at historically high levels both here in the United States and around the globe with questionable benefits. Given this background, the National Institutes of Health, the American College of Obstetricians and Gynecologists and the Society for Maternal-Fetal Medicine convened a consensus conference to work on primary prevention of cesarean delivery. Recommendations from this meeting were summarized in a document published in 2012.[29] Further, the American College of Obstetricians and Gynecologists and the Society for Maternal-Fetal Medicine published an Obstetric Care Consensus document that delineated a number of approaches to safely reducing the cesarean delivery rate.[30] When considering how the cesarean rate might be safely and meaningfully lowered, it is important to consider the most common indications for cesarean delivery, which are a prior cesarean, failed progression in labor, and abnormal fetal heart rate tracing. Potential approaches and frame their potential impact on the cesarean delivery rate are outlined herein.

VAGINAL BIRTH AFTER CESAREAN DELIVERY

Whereas the documents listed focus on the prevention of the primary cesarean, in the one previous time that the cesarean rate was lowered in the United States, the focus was on TOLAC. Unfortunately, a backlash against attempting TOLAC by many hospitals and providers alike has led to a national VBAC rate that is less than 10%.[4] Although many women would not choose to undergo TOLAC, evidence suggests that more than 10% do so and that the current environment is not conducive to achieving a VBAC for many such women. Although VBAC should likely not be universally available at every hospital in the country, there are many hospitals where a safe TOLAC could be offered that do not support TOLAC. Organizational changes in obstetric units such as having laborists available around the clock as well as the availability of in-house anesthesia have improved the safety of a TOLAC, and this remains a viable way to reduce the cesarean delivery rate overall. Even if the VBAC rate increased back up to 25% from the current 10%, there would be far fewer repeat cesarean deliveries.

LABOR MANAGEMENT

The bulk of indicated cesarean deliveries are performed for failed progression of labor during the first or second stages of labor. Labor dystocia has been estimated to account for about one-fifth of all cesarean deliveries.[28] Because the majority of these cesarean deliveries are in women with no prior cesarean delivery, many are primary cesarean deliveries that then lead to future cesarean deliveries because the VBAC rate is so low. The single most common indication is for failed progression in the first stage of labor, commonly diagnosed as active phase arrest. Failed progress in labor is traditionally based on labor norms established more than 50 years ago from a single study.

In 1954, Dr Emmanuel Friedman published a prospective analysis of labor norms drawn from a relatively small cohort of approximately 500 women.[3] This study provided labor thresholds such as the fifth centile of progression (the 95th centile of length of time to achieve 1 cm of dilation) throughout labor.[31] These thresholds became universally accepted and used to ascertain when a labor was going too long. In Friedman's study, the first stage of labor was broken into the latent and active phases, which were commonly demarcated by a cervical dilation of 3 to 4 cm. This threshold identified the beginning of when labor began to progress rapidly. Thus, during the latent phase, it was understood that labor could progress slowly but, once the onset of active labor began, generally, a progression of at least 1 cm of dilation per hour was anticipated. When progress was slower than this, a laboring woman could be said to be "falling off of the labor curve." Given this threshold and with this understanding, when a woman made no progress in the active phase for 2 hours, active phase arrest was diagnosed and became a leading indication for cesarean delivery.

However, recent evidence refutes the use of these thresholds. For example, the largest study of labor, the Consortium on Safe Labor, reported that the 95th centile of progress in labor from 4 to 5 cm is 6.4 hours and from 5 to 6 cm is 3.2 hours.[32] This suggests that the active phase of labor may not begin until 6 cm of dilation in some women and a slow progression from 4 to 6 cm should be tolerated. Furthermore, the 2-hour threshold diagnosis of active phase arrest was challenged by a prospective study.[33] In that study, the authors demonstrated that waiting for cervical change during the active phase of labor for at least 4 hours in the setting of adequate contractions or 6 hours without adequate contractions would lead to 60% of such women going on to deliver vaginally without evidence of harm to either the mother or infant. In a similar study, the investigators found not only would the cesarean rate be reduced and no evidence of increased neonatal morbidity, but the risk of complications in women was lowered.[34]

In the second stage of labor, similarly the amount of time beyond which a second stage of labor was characterized as prolonged has likely been too short. One example of this is that although 1 additional hour of the second stage has been traditionally used for women with an epidural, this seems to have been based on mean or median differences that are generally less than 1 hour.[35] However, when a recent study examined the 95th centile of differences between women without epidural in the second stage, a difference of 2 hours or more was identified in both nulliparous and multiparous women.[36] Thus, management in the second stage of labor should entail ongoing assessment of progress during the second stage, but allowing for at least 2 hours of second stage in multiparous and 3 hours of second stage in nulliparous women, and further allowing for an additional 2 hours in women with an epidural.

In addition to increased patience during the second stage, when the fetal vertex is engaged, operative vaginal delivery remains a beneficial adjunct to achieve vaginal delivery, although it has declined in recent years.[37] Thus, it is important that the next generation of providers continue to be trained to perform operative vaginal deliveries.[38]

ABNORMAL FETAL HEART RATE TRACINGS

After abnormal progression in labor, the second most common indication for a cesarean during labor is an abnormal or indeterminate fetal heart rate tracing. Currently, fetal heart tracings are commonly described as belonging to 1 of 3 categories—I, II, and III. Category I tracings are entirely benign and generally of no concern whatsoever. Category III tracings are almost always an indication for immediate delivery and rarely controversial. However, a large majority of fetal heart rate tracings are described as category II. For example, in 1 recent study, more than 90% of fetal heart rate tracings were category II during the second stage of labor.[39] Category II tracings are labeled indeterminate, although they are not particularly predictive of neonatal acidemia.[40] Thus, category II tracings may have some features of concern, such as fetal heart rate decelerations, but may have other reassuring features such as moderate variability. Thus, in an effort to prevent fetal/neonatal acidemia, many cesarean deliveries are performed for category II fetal heart rate tracings. To avoid unnecessary cesarean deliveries, a variety of intervening steps should be taken before operative delivery is carried out. There are a range of resuscitative measures, such as maternal position change, intravenous fluids, and ensuring adequate blood pressure after obtaining regional analgesia. Additionally, in the setting of repetitive fetal heart rate decelerations, if oxytocin augmentation is being used, this measure can be decreased or halted if there is concern. Another approach for such repetitive decelerations has been the use of intrauterine pressure catheter and amnioinfusion.[41] Finally, if there is not moderate variability to reassure the clinician, fetal scalp stimulation with a response of a fetal heart rate acceleration is quite useful to ensure a pH of greater than 7.20.[42] Despite these approaches, there are still likely too many cesarean deliveries performed for concern about fetal heart rate tracings. Despite the ubiquitous use of continuous fetal heart rate tracings for 40 years, there is a great ongoing need for more clinical research to ascertain the best use of this technology.

MALPOSITION

An additional issue raised about management of patients in the second stage of labor is for those with fetal malposition, in particular, the occiput transverse or occiput posterior positions. It is estimated that persistent fetal malposition occurs in approximately 5% of laboring fetuses, is increased with epidurals, and is associated with an increased risk of cesarean delivery and with both maternal and neonatal complications.[43] One approach to fetal malposition is increased patience in both the first and second stages of labor. Similar to the effect of the epidural on the length of second stage of labor, fetal malposition leads to both longer first and second stages of labor. However, it does seem that fetal malposition cannot always be overcome simply by increasing the length of time in the first or second stage. In the second stage, rotation of the fetal occiput is a useful obstetric skill. Historically, this was accomplished with forceps, particularly the Kielland forceps.[44] However, with a decreasing proportion of providers being trained to perform forceps rotations, increasingly the approach taken is manual rotation of the fetal occiput.[45] This approach has been shown to significantly reduce the risk of cesarean delivery and is relatively safe and easy to train.

MALPRESENTATION

Fetal malpresentation, most commonly breech presentation at term, is seen in approximately 4% of pregnancies.[46] Currently, the vast majority of such pregnancies are delivered via cesarean delivery. Thus, the primary approach to reducing cesarean deliveries in the setting of breech presentation is the use of external cephalic version (ECV) before the onset of labor, usually at 36 to 37 weeks of gestation. In general, ECV is effective in approximately 70% of attempts and the majority of women with a successful ECV go on to deliver vaginally.[47] Additionally, ECV success has been shown to be improved with the use of regional anesthesia; thus, its use would likely reduce cesarean deliveries for malpresentation.[48] Last, moxibustion (a Chinese medicine approach) has been shown to reduce breech presentation and should be at least mentioned to patients with a breech-presenting fetus.[49]

TWIN GESTATIONS

Simply put, there is supportive evidence for attempting vaginal delivery in the setting of a twin gestation with the presenting twin in a cephalic presentation. In particular, a recent randomized trial found no improvement in neonatal outcomes in the setting of planned cesarean for a twin gestation.[50] Thus, continued training of providers to be able to provide vaginal delivery for both vertex–vertex and vertex–breech twins is imperative to allow this option for all women with twin gestations.

INDUCTION OF LABOR

Interestingly, induction of labor has received a lot of negative attention as a source of cesarean deliveries. However, the evidence is not entirely clear regarding induction and cesarean delivery. Although retrospective studies that compare induction of labor and spontaneous labor do find such an association, this is an improper comparison. The true alternative to induction of labor is expectant management as opposed to spontaneous labor.[51] When induction of labor is compared with expectant management, it does not seem to be associated with an increase in the risk of cesarean delivery.[52,53] Further, in prospective, randomized trials at 41 weeks of gestation and beyond, the risk of cesarean delivery is lower in the women who were induced.[54,55]

Given this evidence, one might come to the conclusion that all women should be induced to prevent cesarean deliveries. However, that approach has not been demonstrated in large trials. In fact, routine induction of labor in the wrong setting may increase the risk of cesarean delivery. In particular, if length of time is being used to define a failed induction of labor, that can lead to an increase in cesarean deliveries.[56] Thus, the Safe Prevention of the First Cesarean document suggested that no induction be called a failed induction until at least 24 hours of induction attempt or at least 12 to 18 hours of ruptured membranes. Additionally, induction techniques should include the vast array of cervical ripening agents (eg, prostaglandins, Foley bulb) approaches to the unfavorable cervix.[57]

OTHER MANAGEMENT ISSUES

Another practice that has been found to reduce the rate of cesarean delivery is continuous labor support.[58] Whether the person providing the support needs to have specific training (eg, a doula) or a longstanding relationship with the patient is less clear, but this has led to some institutions creating a doula pool for women who have not arranged for one before labor and delivery. The exact mechanism of labor support in reducing cesarean deliveries is unclear, but it certainly seems to be an inexpensive way to avoid an operative delivery. Another approach is delayed admission in the latent phase of labor. Although there are no randomized trials, 1 study found that the practice reduced cesarean deliveries and saved costs.[59] However, another recent study did not demonstrate a difference from this practice.[60] These management issues are also going to vary based on the local obstetric culture. Any attempt to successfully reduce the rate of cesarean deliveries will likely have to have obstetric culture change as a component.

SUMMARY

Although cesarean delivery may be an increasingly safe alternative to vaginal delivery, its use in 1 in 3 women giving birth is likely too high. Furthermore, the downstream impact of cesarean delivery on future pregnancies is likely not well-considered when the first cesarean delivery is being performed. There are a range of practices that have become standard usage over decades that should be carefully questioned and replaced by standardized, evidence-based practices. In doing so, the rate of cesarean deliveries may be safely decreased. However, given the practice environment that clinicians are facing and the cultural and medicolegal pressures, there will need to be systems approaches that will need to be adopted to affect the cesarean delivery rate at a national level.[61] Through such quality improvement efforts that are health system wide and even statewide, through perinatal quality collaboratives as well as through tort reform efforts, the environmental changes will allow clinicians to adopt the range of practices described. However, without such environmental changes, clinicians may not be able to change their own practice patterns that have been encouraged by the given environments in which they practice.

REFERENCES

1. Neggers YH. Trends in maternal mortality in the United States. Reprod Toxicol 2016;64:72–6.
2. Molina G, Weiser TG, Lipsitz SR, et al. Relationship between cesarean delivery rate and maternal and neonatal mortality. JAMA 2015;314(21):2263–70.
3. Friedman E. The graphic analysis of labor. Am J Obstet Gynecol 1954;68: 1568–75.
4. Martin JA, Hamilton BE, Osterman MJ, et al. Births: final data for 2015. Natl Vital Stat Rep 2017;66(1):1.
5. Menacker F, Hamilton BE. Recent trends in cesarean delivery in the United States. NCHS Data Brief 2010;(35):1–8.
6. U.S. Department of Health and Human Services: Office of Disease Prevention and Health Promotion–Healthy People 2010. Nasnewsletter 2000;15:3.
7. Kozhimannil KB, Law MR, Virnig BA. Cesarean delivery rates vary tenfold among US hospitals; reducing variation may address quality and cost issues. Health Aff (Millwood) 2013;32(3):527–35.
8. Kozhimannil KB, Arcaya MC, Subramanian SV. Maternal clinical diagnoses and hospital variation in the risk of cesarean delivery: analyses of a National US Hospital Discharge Database. PLoS Med 2014;11(10):e1001745.
9. Stotland NE, Caughey AB, Breed E, et al. Macrosomia in a large managed care cohort: maternal risk factors and complications. Int J Gynaecol Obstet 2004;87: 220–6.
10. Weiss JL, Malone FD, Emig D, et al. Obesity, obstetric complications and cesarean delivery rate–a population-based screening study. Am J Obstet Gynecol 2004;190:1091–7.
11. Stotland NE, Hopkins LM, Caughey AB. Gestational weight gain, macrosomia, and the risk of cesarean birth. Obstet Gynecol 2004;104:671–7.
12. Ogden CL, Carroll MD, Curtin LR, et al. Prevalence of overweight and obesity in the United States, 1999-2004. JAMA 2006;295(13):1549–55.

13. Marshall NE, Guild C, Cheng YW, et al. Maternal super-obesity and perinatal outcomes. Am J Obstet Gynecol 2012;206(5):417.e1-6.
14. Swank ML, Caughey AB, Farinelli CK, et al. The impact of change in pregnancy body mass index on cesarean delivery. J Matern Fetal Neonatal Med 2014;27(8): 795–800.
15. Meikle SF, Steiner CA, Zhang J, et al. A national estimate of the elective primary cesarean delivery rate. Obstet Gynecol 2005;105:751–6.
16. Angeja A, Caughey AB, Vargas J, et al. Chilean women's preferences regarding mode of delivery: which do they prefer and why? Obstet Gynecol 2004;103:117S.
17. National Institutes of Health. Cesarean Delivery on Maternal Request. State-of-the-Science Conference Statement. Obstet Gynecol 2006;107(6):1386–97.
18. Sparks TN, Yeaton-Massey A, Granados JM, et al. Preference toward future mode of delivery: how do antepartum preferences and prior delivery experience contribute? J Matern Fetal Neonatal Med 2015;28(14):1673–8.
19. Cheng YW, Snowden JM, Handler SJ, et al. Litigation in obstetrics: does defensive medicine contribute to increases in cesarean delivery? J Matern Fetal Neonatal Med 2014;27(16):1668–75.
20. Yang YT, Mello MM, Subramanian SV, et al. Relationship between malpractice litigation pressure and rates of cesarean section and vaginal birth after cesarean section. Med Care 2009;47(2):234–42.
21. Minkoff H, Chervenak FA. Elective primary cesarean delivery. N Engl J Med 2003; 348:946–50.
22. Harper MA, Byington RP, Espeland MA, et al. Pregnancy-related death and health care services. Obstet Gynecol 2003;102(2):273–8.
23. Handa VL, Harris TA, Ostergard DR. Protecting the pelvic floor: obstetric management to prevent incontinence and pelvic organ prolapse. Obstet Gynecol 1996;88:470–8.
24. Landon MB, Hauth JC, Leveno KJ, et al. Maternal and perinatal outcomes associated with a trial of labor after prior cesarean delivery. N Engl J Med 2004;351: 2581–9.
25. Silver RM, Landon MB, Rouse DJ, et al. Maternal morbidity associated with multiple repeat cesarean deliveries. Obstet Gynecol 2006;107(6):1226–32.
26. Solheim K, Esakoff TF, Little SE, et al. The effect of current cesarean delivery rates on the future incidence of placenta previa, placenta accreta, and maternal mortality. J Matern Fetal Neonatal Med 2011;24:1341–6.
27. Smith GC, Pell JP, Cameron AD, et al. Risk of Perinatal death associated with labor after previous cesarean delivery in uncomplicated term pregnancies. JAMA 2002;287:2684–90.
28. Smith GC, Pell JP, Dobbie R. Caesarean section and risk of unexplained stillbirth in subsequent pregnancy. Lancet 2003;362:1779–84.
29. Spong CY, Berghella V, Wenstrom KD, et al. Preventing the first cesarean delivery: summary of a joint Eunice Kennedy Shriver National Institute of Child Health and Human Development, Society for Maternal-Fetal Medicine, and American College of Obstetricians and Gynecologists Workshop. Obstet Gynecol 2012; 120(5):1181–93.
30. American College of Obstetricians and Gynecologists (College), Society for Maternal-Fetal Medicine, Caughey AB, Cahill AG, Guise J-M, et al. Safe prevention of the primary cesarean delivery. Obstetric Consensus Document. Am J Obstet Gynecol 2014;210(3):179–93.
31. Friedman EA. An objective approach to the diagnosis and management of abnormal labor. Bull N Y Acad Med 1972;48:842–58.

32. Zhang J, Landy HJ, Branch W, et al. Contemporary patterns of spontaneous labor with normal neonatal outcomes. Obstet Gynecol 2010;116:1281–7.

33. Rouse DJ, Owen J, Savage K, et al. Active phase labor arrest: revisiting the 2-hour minimum. Obstet Gynecol 2001;98(4):550–4.

34. Henry DM, Cheng YW, Shaffer BL, et al. Perinatal outcomes in active phase arrest and vaginal delivery. Obstet Gynecol 2008;112:1109–15.

35. Kilpatrick SJ, Laros RK Jr. Characteristics of normal labor. Obstet Gynecol 1989; 74(1):85–7.

36. Cheng YW, Shaffer BL, Nicholson JM, et al. Second stage of labor and epidural use: a larger effect than previously suggested. Obstet Gynecol 2014;123(3): 527–35.

37. Srinivas SK, Epstein AJ, Nicholson S, et al. Improvements in US maternal obstetrical outcomes from 1992 to 2006. Med Care 2010;48(5):487–93.

38. Shaffer BL, Caughey AB. Forceps delivery: potential benefits and a call for continued training. J Perinatol 2007;27:327–8.

39. Cahill AG, Roehl KA, Odibo AO, et al. Association and prediction of neonatal acidemia. Am J Obstet Gynecol 2012;207:206.e1-8.

40. Cahill AG, Roehl KA, Odibo AO, et al. Association of atypical decelerations with acidemia. Obstet Gynecol 2012;120:1387–93.

41. Macri CJ, Schrimmer DB, Leung A, et al. Prophylactic amnioinfusion improves outcome of pregnancy complicated by thick meconium and oligohydramnios. Am J Obstet Gynecol 1992;167:117–21.

42. Elimian A, Figueroa R, Tejani N. Intrapartum assessment of fetal well-being: a comparison of scalp stimulation with scalp blood pH sampling. Obstet Gynecol 1997;89:373–6.

43. Cheng YW, Hubbard A, Caughey AB, et al. Use of propensity scores to estimate the effect of persistent occiput posterior on perinatal outcomes. Am J Epidemiol 2010;171:656–63.

44. Nash Z, Nathan B, Mascarenhas L. Kielland's forceps. From controversy to consensus? Acta Obstet Gynecol Scand 2015;94(1):8–12.

45. Shaffer BL, Cheng YW, Vargas J, et al. Manual rotation of the fetal occiput in persistent transverse or posterior positions. J Matern Fetal Neonatal Med 2011; 24:65–72.

46. Lee HC, El-Sayed YY, Gould JB. Population trends in cesarean delivery for breech presentation in the United States, 1997-2003. Am J Obstet Gynecol 2008;199:59.e1-8.

47. Clock C, Kurtzman J, White J, et al. Cesarean risk after successful external cephalic version: a matched, retrospective analysis. J Perinatol 2009;29:96–100.

48. Yoshida M, Matsuda H, Kawakami Y, et al. Effectiveness of epidural anesthesia for external cephalic version (ECV). J Perinatol 2010;30:580–3.

49. Cardini F, Weixin H. Moxibustion for correction of breech presentation: a randomized controlled trial. JAMA 1998;280(18):1580–4.

50. Barrett JF, Hannah ME, Hutton EK, et al, Twin Birth Study Collaborative Group. A randomized trial of planned cesarean or vaginal delivery for twin pregnancy. N Engl J Med 2013;369(14):1295–305.

51. Caughey AB, Nicholson JM, Cheng YW, et al. Induction of labor and cesarean delivery by gestational age. Am J Obstet Gynecol 2006;195:700–5.

52. Darney BG, Snowden JM, Cheng YW, et al. Elective induction of labor at term compared to expectant management: maternal and neonatal outcomes. Obstet Gynecol 2013;122:1–10.

53. Stock SJ, Ferguson E, Duffy A, et al. Outcomes of elective induction of labour compared with expectant management: population based study. BMJ 2012; 344:e2838.
54. Gulmezoglu AM, Crowther CA, Middleton P, et al. Induction of labour for improving birth outcomes for women at or beyond term. Cochrane Database Syst Rev 2012;(6):CD004945.
55. Caughey AB, Sundaram V, Kaimal A, et al. Elective Induction of labor vs. expectant management of pregnancy: a systematic review. Ann Intern Med 2009;151: 252–63.
56. Rouse DJ, Owen J, Hauth JC. Criteria for failed labor induction: prospective evaluation of a standardized protocol. Obstet Gynecol 2000;96:671–7.
57. Wing DA, Sheibani L. Pharmacotherapy options for labor induction. Expert Opin Pharmacother 2015;16(11):1657–68.
58. Hodnett ED, Gates S, Hofmeyr GJ, et al. Continuous support for women during childbirth. Cochrane Database Syst Rev 2012;(10):CD003766.
59. Tilden EL, Lee VR, Allen AJ, et al. Cost-effectiveness analysis of latent versus active labor hospital admission for medically low-risk, term women. Birth 2015; 42(3):219–26.
60. Nelson DB, McIntire DD, Leveno KJ. False labor at term in singleton pregnancies: discharge after a standardized assessment and perinatal outcomes. Obstet Gynecol 2017;130(1):139–45.
61. Cheng YW, Snowden JM, Handler S, et al. Clinicians' practice environment is associated with a higher likelihood of recommending cesarean deliveries. J Matern Fetal Neonatal Med 2014;27(12):1220–7.

Defining and Managing Normal and Abnormal First Stage of Labor

Janine S. Rhoades, MD, Alison G. Cahill, MD, MSCI*

KEYWORDS

- First stage of labor • Labor • Labor arrest • Labor curve • Labor dystocia

KEY POINTS

- The first stage of labor has a significantly longer latent phase than was previously thought, especially in nulliparous patients, obese patients, and induction of labor.
- The transition from the latent phase to the active phase of labor does not occur until 6 cm of cervical dilatation in all patients.
- Arrest of the first stage of labor is diagnosed by greater than or equal to 6 cm of dilatation, ruptured membranes, and no cervical change with 4 hours of adequate or 6 hours of inadequate contractions.
- Failed induction of labor is diagnosed after cervical ripening by failure to generate regular contractions and cervical change with 24 hours of oxytocin and rupture of membranes.
- Providers should be aware of abnormal progression in the first stage of labor and use oxytocin, internal tocodynamometry, and/or amniotomy to increase the likelihood of vaginal delivery.

INTRODUCTION

There has been a dramatic increase in the cesarean delivery (CD) rate over the past 15 years. CD is the most common major surgery performed in the United States and approximately 1 of every 3 pregnancies is delivered by CD. In 2007, 26.5% of low-risk primiparous patients had a CD. Of US women who require an initial cesarean, more than 90% have a subsequent repeat CD.[1]

Given that 90% of women have a repeat CD, the most effective approach to reducing the cesarean rate and its associated morbidities is to reduce the primary CD rate. The first step to reduce the primary CD rate is to assess the indications for which primary cesareans are performed. A recent study found that a diagnosis of labor arrest accounted for the largest portion of primary CD at 34% (**Fig. 1**).[2] This large

Disclosure: The authors report no conflicts of interest.
Department of Obstetrics and Gynecology, Washington University in St. Louis, 660 South Euclid Avenue, Campus Box 8064, St Louis, MO 63110, USA
* Corresponding author.
E-mail address: cahilla@wudosis.wustl.edu

Obstet Gynecol Clin N Am 44 (2017) 535–545
http://dx.doi.org/10.1016/j.ogc.2017.07.001
0889-8545/17/© 2017 Elsevier Inc. All rights reserved.

obgyn.theclinics.com

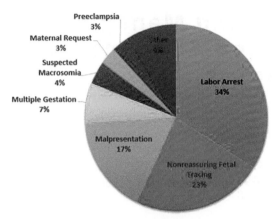

Fig. 1. Indications for primary CD. (*Adapted from* Barber EL, Lundsberg LS, Belanger K, et al. Indications contributing to the increasing cesarean delivery rate. Obstet Gynecol 2011;118(1):29–38; with permission.)

contribution to the primary CD rate is potentially modifiable with appropriate management of labor and diagnosis of labor arrest.

This article reviews the normal progression of the first stage of labor for patients in spontaneous labor as well as several special populations, defines labor arrest in the modern obstetric population, and discusses management options for abnormal first stage of labor progression.

HISTORIC VERSUS MODERN LABOR CURVE

Until recently, the definition of normal first-stage labor progression was based on data published in the 1950s. The traditional Friedman labor curve described the latent phase of labor from 0 to 4 cm, at which point the slope of the curve increased with more rapid cervical change in the active phase of labor from 4 to 10 cm. Friedman[3] also described a deceleration phase as the patient reached 9 to 10 cm, at which point labor progression slowed (**Fig. 2**).

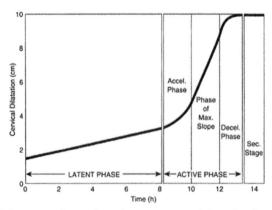

Fig. 2. Historical labor curve for patients in spontaneous labor. Accel, acceleration; Decel, deceleration; Max, maximum; Sec, second. (*Adapted from* Friedman EA. The graphic analysis of labor. Am J Obstet Gynecol 1954;68(6):1572; with permission.)

In contrast, the modern labor curve identifies a transition from the latent to active phase of labor at about 6 cm of cervical dilatation. Before 6 cm, the latent phase of labor is longer and progresses more slowly than that described by Friedman.[3] However, the active phase of labor progresses more quickly, especially in multiparous patients. In the modern curve, there is no deceleration phase near 10 cm (**Fig. 3**).[4]

The differences in these 2 labor curves are attributable to many factors. First, the obstetric patient population is drastically different now from that of the 1950s. Obstetric patients now are generally older, of greater maternal weight, have increased use of anesthesia in labor, increased use of induction or augmentation of labor, and deliver babies of higher birth weight compared with patients in the 1950s. In addition, the updated labor curve was constructed using modern statistical methods that account for cervical examinations being repeated many times in the same patient, and for the impossibility of knowing at exactly what time a patient's cervix changed from 1 cm to the next.[4]

SPONTANEOUS LABOR

In 2010, Zhang and colleagues[4] published data on the normal progression of spontaneous labor in a contemporary patient cohort. They included more than 60,000 patients from 19 hospitals across the United States with term pregnancies who achieved a vaginal delivery with normal neonatal outcomes. They stratified their analysis by parity. Nulliparous and multiparous women progressed similarly in labor up to 6 cm of cervical dilatation. In this latent phase of labor, they found that it may take more than 7 hours to progress from 4 to 5 cm and more than 3 hours to progress from 5 to 6 cm, regardless of parity. After 6 cm, labor progressed more rapidly, especially in multiparous women, indicating the active phase of labor. In the active phase of labor, they found that it may take 1.4 to 2.2 hours to progress each centimeter for nulliparous patients and 0.8 to 1.8 hours for multiparous patients. These data allowed construction of the modern labor curve described previously of the expected normal progression of the first stage of labor for patients in spontaneous labor.

Using the modern definitions of spontaneous labor, Wood and colleagues[5] assessed the optimal cervical dilatation for admission of women in spontaneous labor with intact membranes at term. They assessed the risk of CD based on more than 2000 patients' cervical dilatation on admission for spontaneous labor. Admission in latent labor at less than 6 cm was associated with an increased risk of CD compared

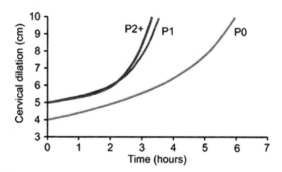

Fig. 3. Modern labor curve for patients in spontaneous labor stratified by parity. P0, nulliparous; P1, parity of 1; P2+, parity of 2 or greater. (*From* Zhang J, Landy HJ, Branch DW, et al. Contemporary patterns of spontaneous labor with normal neonatal outcomes. Obstet Gynecol 2010;116(6):1283; with permission.)

with women admitted at greater than or equal to 6 cm (13.2% vs 3.5%; relative risk, 3.73; 95% confidence interval, 1.94, 7.17). They analyzed each individual centimeter of cervical dilatation, and there was a higher rate of cesarean and cesarean for labor arrest at each centimeter of admission cervical dilatation less than 5 cm (**Fig. 4**).[5] Based on these data, it may be prudent to consider deferring admission of patients with intact membranes in latent labor at term to decrease their risk of CD, especially patients who are less than 5 cm dilated.

INDUCED LABOR

Induction of labor has become increasingly common and has increased 140% since 1990.[6] Several studies have associated induction of labor with an increased risk of CD.[7–9] However, many of these studies have compared patients who were induced with those in spontaneous labor at the same gestational age. This comparison is unfair because the alternative to an induction of labor is ongoing expectant management of the pregnancy, not spontaneous labor. In addition, an induction of labor is a different process compared with a woman who presents in spontaneous labor, and the definitions of normal spontaneous labor cannot be directly applied to induced labor.

In order to define normal progression of induced labor, Harper and colleagues[6] conducted a study of more than 5000 term pregnancies that reached 10 cm of cervical dilatation. They compared normal labor progression in women whose labor was induced with women whose labor was spontaneous and stratified by parity. The median time to progress from 4 to 10 cm in induced nulliparous patients was 5.5 hours; however, it may take as long as nearly 17 hours (95th percentile). This time is significantly longer than the time for nulliparous patients in spontaneous labor to progress from 4 to 10 cm (median, 3.8 hours; 95th percentile, 11.8 hours). Their findings were similar in multiparous patients. The median time to progress from 4 to 10 cm was 4.4 hours for induced multiparous patients, with an upper limit of normal of 16.2 hours. In comparison, multiparous patients in spontaneous labor had a median of 2.4 hours to progress from 4 to 10 cm with a 95th percentile of 8.8 hours. For both nulliparous

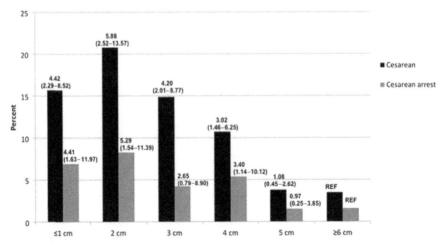

Fig. 4. Relative risk of CD based on admission cervical dilatation of patients in spontaneous labor. (*From* Wood AM, Frey HA, Tuuli MG, et al. Optimal admission cervical dilation in spontaneously laboring women. Am J Perinatol 2016;33(2):190; with permission.)

and multiparous patients, once women reached the active phase of labor (6 cm or greater), both induced and spontaneous labor progressed at similar rates.

Overall, regardless of parity, induced labor has a significantly longer latent phase than spontaneous labor. However, the active phase of labor is similar between the two groups. The previously described increased rate of CD in patients who undergo induction of labor is likely at least in part caused by providers inappropriately holding induced patients to the same standard of expected labor progression as patients in spontaneous labor, which leads to a premature diagnosis of labor arrest in the latent phase of induced labor.

SPECIAL POPULATIONS

There are several unique populations for whom a normal first stage of labor may be slightly different from that of the general population. Three such populations that have been studied are discussed later: obese patients, patients in preterm labor, and patients undergoing a trial of labor after cesarean (TOLAC).

OBESITY

Obesity is an independent risk factor for CD and the complications of CD, such as wound separation or infection, anesthetic complications, and thrombosis, disproportionately affect obese women. To characterize normal progression of the first stage of labor in obese women, Norman and colleagues[10] conducted a study of more than 5000 women at term who reached 10 cm of cervical dilatation. They compared labor progression between obese (body mass index [BMI] $\geq$30 kg/m^2) and nonobese (BMI <30 kg/m^2) patients. The median time for obese patients to progress from 4 to 10 cm was significantly longer than for nonobese patients (4.7 hours vs 4.1 hours; P<.01). In addition, the upper limit of normal (95th percentile) was more than 16 hours for obese patients compared with 14 hours for nonobese patients. These differences were most notable in the latent phase of labor. After 6 cm of cervical dilatation, there was no longer a significant difference in the rate of progression. These findings were consistent for both nulliparous and multiparous patients (**Fig. 5**).

When their results were stratified by BMI 30 to 40 kg/m^2 and BMI greater than 40 kg/m^2, increasing BMI was associated with a significantly longer time to reach

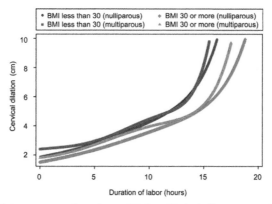

Fig. 5. Average labor curves for obese (BMI $\geq$30 kg/m^2) compared with nonobese (BMI <30 kg/m^2) patients stratified by parity. (*From* Norman SM, Tuuli MG, Odibo AO, et al. The effects of obesity on the first stage of labor. Obstet Gynecol 2012;120(1):133; with permission.)

each centimeter of cervical dilatation up to 6 cm. In addition, the median time to progress from 4 to 10 cm was approximately 2 hours longer in patients with BMI greater than 40 kg/m^2 than in normal-weight patients (BMI, 25 kg/m^2 or less) for both nulliparous (6.7 hours vs 4.6 hours) and multiparous (5.0 hours vs 3.3 hours) women. Strikingly, the 95th percentile for time to progress from 4 to 10 cm for patients with BMI greater than 40 kg/m^2 was 21.2 hours for nulliparous patients (compared with 14.4 hours for normal-weight patients) and 19.2 hours for multiparous patients (compared with 12.6 hours for normal-weight patients).[10]

In summary, maternal obesity significantly prolongs the normal first stage of labor, particularly the latent phase of labor, even in multiparous patients. As the severity of obesity increases, the effect on prolonging the first stage of labor is more notable. Thus, it is prudent for providers to consider the patient's BMI when interpreting the patient's labor curve and considering a diagnosis of labor arrest.

PRETERM LABOR

Preterm labor is common; approximately 1 of every 8 infants in the United States is born preterm (<37 weeks' gestational age). However, patients who deliver preterm were excluded from both historical and modern studies of normal labor progression. To define normal progression in preterm labor, Spain and colleagues[11] compared the first stage of preterm labor with the first stage of term labor in a cohort of more than 5000 births greater than or equal to 24 weeks' gestation who reached 10 cm of cervical dilatation. The median time to progress from 4 to 10 cm was significantly faster in preterm labor than in term labor, and this was true for both nulliparous and multiparous patients, as well as patients in induced or spontaneous labor. The primary difference in the labor curves between preterm and term labor was in the active phase of labor when preterm labor progressed more rapidly than term labor. Importantly, the transition from latent to active labor occurred at about 6 cm of cervical dilatation, similar to patients in labor at term. These data on the normal labor curve for the first stage of preterm labor are clinically useful for understanding the expected labor progression in patients undergoing an indicated preterm delivery, as well as for determining the stability of patients in preterm labor for transport to a tertiary care facility.

TRIAL OF LABOR AFTER CESAREAN

Another unique population to consider are those laboring patients who have undergone a previous CD. Graseck and colleagues[12] compared the first stage of term, spontaneous labor, in patients undergoing trial of labor after cesarean (TOLAC) with those without a history of CD. They included more than 2000 patients who reached 10 cm of cervical dilatation. They found no difference in the rate of cervical dilatation between patients undergoing TOLAC and the non-TOLAC group. The investigators stratified their analysis by a history of a previous vaginal delivery and found no change in their results. Thus, the expected progression in the first stage of spontaneous labor for patients undergoing TOLAC is the same as for those patients without a prior cesarean. The diagnosis of labor arrest should be made by the same criteria as for patients without a uterine scar.

An additional study by Sondgeroth and colleagues[13] included 473 patients with a prior CD who achieved a vaginal birth after cesarean at term and compared the first stage of labor between those patients who were induced and those who had spontaneous labor. Similar to previous data from patients without a uterine scar, patients induced with a prior CD progressed more slowly in the first stage of labor than patients in spontaneous labor with a prior CD. This difference was most notable in the latent phase of labor and the progression was similar between the 2 groups in the active phase of labor after 6 cm of cervical dilatation. Patients undergoing an induction of labor with a history of a CD should be expected to progress in the first stage of labor similarly to those patients who are induced without a prior CD with a significantly longer latent phase of labor than patients in spontaneous labor.

FETAL DESCENT

In addition to cervical dilatation, fetal descent within the pelvis is also necessary to reach a vaginal delivery and is another important consideration when assessing a patient's progress in the first stage of labor. In order to define normal fetal descent in the first stage of labor, Graseck and colleagues[14] conducted a retrospective cohort study of more than 4500 term patients who achieved a vaginal delivery and determined the duration of labor between levels of station and estimated the median station for each given cervical dilatation. They stratified their analysis by parity and by spontaneous or induced labor.

The investigators found that multiparous women had faster fetal descent than nulliparous women at all stations except from +2 to +3 station when descent was similar to nulliparous patients. Similarly, women in spontaneous labor had faster fetal descent than women whose labor was induced or augmented at all stations except +2 to +3 when again the duration was comparable between the 2 groups. The investigators noted that there was wide variation in the normal length of time spent at high station (>0 station), especially in nulliparous and induced patients. The 95th percentile included more than 12 hours for nulliparous patients to descend from −2 to −1 station.

In general, multiparous women had a higher station at greater cervical dilatation than nulliparous women. However, 95% of all patients were 0 station or lower at 10 cm of cervical dilatation.[14] Providers should be comfortable with slow descent from high stations early in the first stage of labor. However, by complete cervical dilatation a high fetal station should be considered abnormal.

DEFINITIONS OF LABOR ARREST

A workshop was held in 2012 with experts from the Society for Maternal-Fetal Medicine, Eunice Kennedy Shriver National Institute of Child Health and Human Development, and the American College of Obstetricians and Gynecologists to identify strategies to reduce the CD rate, especially the primary cesarean rate.[1] One major focus of this workshop was to redefine recommendations for labor management and diagnosis of labor arrest disorders based on the data on normal modern labor curves.

FIRST-STAGE LABOR ARREST

The traditional definitions of abnormal labor progression and labor arrest were based on the historical labor curve by Friedman.[3] Abnormal labor progression was defined as less than 1.2 cm cervical dilatation per hour in nulliparous patients and less than 1.5 cm/h in multiparous patients. Arrest of the first stage of labor was diagnosed after no cervical change for greater than or equal to 2 hours with adequate contractions and cervical dilatation of at least 4 cm. These definitions are no longer acceptable for use.

The current definition of the first stage of labor arrest requires the patient to (1) be at least 6 cm dilated, (2) have membranes ruptured, and (3) make no cervical change for at least 4 hours of adequate contractions or at least 6 hours of inadequate contractions with oxytocin use to attempt to achieve adequate contractions.[1] Because the active phase of labor does not begin until 6 cm of cervical dilatation, the standards for the active phase labor progress cannot be applied at lesser cervical dilatations and a diagnosis of arrest of the first stage of labor cannot be made until that point. It is also important to note that the term protracted labor is no longer in use. Slow, but progressive, labor should not be an indication for cesarean. In addition, a prolonged latent phase of labor (previously defined as >20 hours in nulliparous patients and >14 hours in multiparous patients) is no longer an indication for CD.[1,15]

FAILED INDUCTION OF LABOR

Before active labor, the diagnosis of arrest of the first stage of labor cannot be made. In that case, the diagnosis is a failed induction of labor. The diagnosis of failed induction of labor requires that the patient (1) has first undergone complete cervical ripening, and then (2) fails to generate regular (every 3 minutes) contractions and cervical change after at least 24 hours of oxytocin with artificial rupture of membranes if possible. A normal induction of labor may take many hours to days and has been associated with an increased risk of CD. Thus it is not recommended to induce a patient with an unfavorable cervix before 41 weeks' gestation unless it is medically indicated. When an induction is indicated with an unfavorable cervix, cervical ripening agents should be used and have been shown to lead to lower rates of cesarean.[1,15]

MANAGEMENT OF ABNORMAL LABOR

A long first stage of labor introduces both maternal and neonatal risk. A retrospective study by Harper and colleagues[16] of more than 5000 women who reached the second stage of labor at term assessed the maternal and neonatal risk associated with increasing duration of the first stage of labor. They compared outcomes in patients whose first stage of labor was less than the 90th percentile, 90th to 94th percentile, 95th to 96th percentile, and greater than or equal to the 97th percentile. Increasing duration of the first stage of labor was associated with an increased risk of maternal fever, shoulder dystocia, and neonatal admission to a level 2 or 3 nursery.

There are several strategies to actively manage the first stage of labor when it begins to progress abnormally. Providers should closely follow each patient's labor curve and be aware of when labor is not progressing as expected. In those situations, the provider should have a low threshold to use interventions such as oxytocin, internal tocodynamometry, and amniotomy to maximize the likelihood of achieving a vaginal delivery.

OXYTOCIN

Oxytocin is the most commonly used intervention for labor dystocia. In a study by Rouse and colleagues,[17] patients in spontaneous labor were initiated on oxytocin augmentation after labor arrest in the active phase. The vaginal delivery rate for multiparous patients who made progress after 2 hours of oxytocin was 99% and for those who made progress after 4 hours of oxytocin it was 98%. Even for those multiparous patients who had not yet made cervical change after 4 hours of oxytocin, 88% still ultimately achieved a vaginal delivery. The results were similar for nulliparous patients. Nulliparas who made progress after 2 hours of oxytocin had a vaginal delivery rate of 97% and those who made cervical change after 4 hours of oxytocin had a vaginal delivery rate of 94%. For those nulliparous patients who had not made labor progress after 4 hours of oxytocin, the vaginal delivery rate was still 56%. There were no severe adverse maternal or neonatal outcomes with the use of oxytocin. Thus, oxytocin is a safe and effective intervention for abnormal progression in the first stage of labor. Administration of oxytocin should be considered a first-line therapy for patients with abnormal progression in the first stage of labor.

INTERNAL TOCODYNAMOMETRY

Internal tocodynamometry by an intrauterine pressure catheter (IUPC) is often used as a means to more accurately quantify the frequency, duration, and magnitude of uterine contractions compared with external tocodynamometry. A randomized controlled trial was conducted in the Netherlands comparing the operative delivery rates (CD or operative vaginal delivery) between patients randomized to receive an IUPC or external tocodynamometry at the beginning of labor. There was no difference in operative delivery rate between the two groups, and no difference in adverse maternal or neonatal outcomes.[18]

Despite no evidence that use of an IUPC reduces the CD rate, its use is advocated by many clinicians. It is not recommended for routine use on all laboring patients, but it is recommended in many special circumstances. One such circumstance is maternal obesity or any other condition in which the external tocodynamometry is not able to accurately record uterine activity. In addition, its use should be strongly considered when a patient is not making expected progress in labor or is not responding as expected to oxytocin augmentation. These special situations have not been specifically studied in trials and these patients likely benefit from the use of an IUPC. Furthermore, in order to diagnose arrest of the first stage of labor, the provider must know whether the patient has adequate or inadequate contractions. The adequacy of contractions can only be determined with an IUPC by calculation of Montevideo units. Thus, for patients who have abnormal progression in the first stage of labor, the use of an IUPC is recommended to assess the patient's response to oxytocin and to determine the adequacy of uterine contractions.

AMNIOTOMY

Artificial rupture of the amniotic membranes (amniotomy) is another commonly used method to augment an abnormal first stage of labor. A randomized controlled trial of nulliparous women in spontaneous labor found that early amniotomy reduced the median length of time to progress to complete cervical dilatation and reduced the rate of labor dystocia. There was no difference in maternal or neonatal outcomes, including infectious outcomes.[19] Although this study did not find a decreased rate of CD with early amniotomy, another recent randomized controlled trial of a similar patient population did find that early amniotomy was associated with a lower rate of labor dystocia as well as CD.[20] A recent Cochrane Review assessed the use of oxytocin and amniotomy in combination compared with expectant management for prevention of, or therapy for, delay in first stage of spontaneous labor progress. The results showed that intervention is associated with a shortened duration of labor and a modest reduction in the rate of CD. Again, no difference was found in adverse maternal or neonatal outcomes.[21] Thus, the combination of oxytocin and amniotomy is safe and effective in the case of abnormal spontaneous labor progression.

SUMMARY

Modern data have redefined the normal first stage of labor and allowed new diagnostic criteria to be established to diagnose first-stage labor arrest and failed induction of labor. Key differences include that the latent phase of labor is much slower than was previously thought and the transition from latent to active labor does not occur until about 6 cm of cervical dilatation, regardless of parity or whether labor was spontaneous or induced.

Diagnosis of arrest of the first stage of labor is only made once the patient is at least 6 cm dilated, has ruptured membranes, and has made no cervical change with 4 hours of adequate contractions or 6 hours of inadequate contractions. Diagnosis of a failed induction of labor is made after the patient has undergone complete cervical ripening, and then has failure to generate regular contractions and cervical change after at least 24 hours of oxytocin with rupture of membranes. Providers should have a low threshold to use one of the known safe and effective interventions to manage the patient with abnormal progression in the first stage of labor, including oxytocin, internal tocodynamometry, and amniotomy.

It is imperative that providers adhere to the new standards for normal progression of the first stage of labor and diagnosis of labor arrest and failed induction of labor in their clinical practices. Labor arrest is the most common indication for a primary CD and there is great potential to decrease the number of cesareans performed for labor arrest with these new diagnostic criteria. This practice has the potential to significantly affect the increasing CD rate and its associated morbidities in the United States.

REFERENCES

1. Spong CY, Berghella V, Wenstrom KD, et al. Preventing the first cesarean delivery: summary of a joint Eunice Kennedy Shriver National Institute of Child Health and Human Development, Society for Maternal-Fetal Medicine, and American College of Obstetricians and Gynecologists workshop. Obstet Gynecol 2012; 120(5):1181–93.
2. Barber EL, Lundsberg LS, Belanger K, et al. Indications contributing to the increasing cesarean delivery rate. Obstet Gynecol 2011;118(1):29–38.
3. Friedman E. The graphic analysis of labor. Am J Obstet Gynecol 1954;68(6): 1568–75.
4. Zhang J, Landy HJ, Branch DW, et al. Contemporary patterns of spontaneous labor with normal neonatal outcomes. Obstet Gynecol 2010;116(6):1281–7.
5. Wood AM, Frey HA, Tuuli MG, et al. Optimal admission cervical dilation in spontaneously laboring women. Am J Perinatol 2016;33(2):188–94.
6. Harper LM, Caughey AB, Odibo AO, et al. Normal progress of induced labor. Obstet Gynecol 2012;119(6):1113–8.
7. Cammu H, Martens G, Ruyssinck G, et al. Outcome after elective labor induction in nulliparous women: a matched cohort study. Am J Obstet Gynecol 2002; 186(2):240–4.
8. Maslow AS, Sweeny AL. Elective induction of labor as a risk factor for cesarean delivery among low-risk women at term. Obstet Gynecol 2000;95(6 Pt 1):917–22.
9. Yeast JD, Jones A, Poskin M. Induction of labor and the relationship to cesarean delivery: A review of 7001 consecutive inductions. Am J Obstet Gynecol 1999; 180(3 Pt 1):628–33.
10. Norman SM, Tuuli MG, Odibo AO, et al. The effects of obesity on the first stage of labor. Obstet Gynecol 2012;120(1):130–5.
11. Spain JE, Tuuli M, Caughey AB, et al. Normal first stage of preterm labor. Am J Perinatol 2014;31(4):315–20.
12. Graseck AS, Odibo AO, Tuuli M, et al. Normal first stage of labor in women undergoing trial of labor after cesarean delivery. Obstet Gynecol 2012;119(4):732–6.
13. Sondgeroth KE, Stout MJ, Graseck AS, et al. Progress of induced labor in trial of labor after cesarean delivery. Am J Obstet Gynecol 2015;213(3):420.e1–5.

14. Graseck A, Tuuli M, Roehl K, et al. Fetal descent in labor. Obstet Gynecol 2014; 123(3):521–6.
15. Caughey AB, Cahill AG, Guise JM, et al. Safe prevention of the primary cesarean delivery. Am J Obstet Gynecol 2014;210(3):179–93.
16. Harper LM, Caughey AB, Roehl KA, et al. Defining an abnormal first stage of labor based on maternal and neonatal outcomes. Am J Obstet Gynecol 2014; 210(6):536.e1–7.
17. Rouse DJ, Owen J, Hauth JC. Active-phase labor arrest: oxytocin augmentation for at least 4 hours. Obstet Gynecol 1999;93(3):323–8.
18. Bakker JJ, Verhoeven CJ, Janssen PF, et al. Outcomes after internal versus external tocodynamometry for monitoring labor. N Engl J Med 2010;362(4): 306–13.
19. Fraser WD, Marcoux S, Moutquin JM, et al. Effect of early amniotomy on the risk of dystocia in nulliparous women. The Canadian Early Amniotomy Study Group. N Engl J Med 1993;328(16):1145–9.
20. Ghafarzadeh M, Moeininasab S, Namdari M. Effect of early amniotomy on dystocia risk and cesarean delivery in nulliparous women: a randomized clinical trial. Arch Gynecol Obstet 2015;292(2):321–5.
21. Wei S, Wo BL, Qi HP, et al. Early amniotomy and early oxytocin for prevention of, or therapy for, delay in first stage spontaneous labour compared with routine care. Cochrane database Syst Rev 2013;(8):CD006794.

Defining and Managing Normal and Abnormal Second Stage of Labor

Yvonne W. Cheng, MD, PhD[a,b,]*, Aaron B. Caughey, MD, PhD[c]

KEYWORDS

- Second stage of labor • Length of labor • Epidural • Cesarean

KEY POINTS

- The norms of the length of the second stage are based on outdated information and appear to be longer than previously thought.
- Interventions in the second stage, such as operative vaginal delivery and cesarean delivery, have unclear benefit and would benefit from carefully designed prospective studies.
- The association between prolonged second stage of labor and neonatal outcomes is not consistent in the literature.
- The association between prolonged second stage of labor and maternal outcomes may be due, in part, to the increased interventions with operative vaginal and cesarean delivery.

INTRODUCTION

Management of the second stage of labor is commonly based on its length such that when second stage exceeds a specific time threshold, women are often counseled and offered potential interventions, including operative vaginal delivery or cesarean delivery due to a "prolonged second stage." In this article, the authors review the basis for defining normal and abnormal length of second stage and discuss the impact of epidural analgesia on the second stage of labor and management of second stage with associated maternal and neonatal outcomes.

Disclosure Statement: The authors have no financial relationship with a company that has any relationship with the content of the article.
[a] Division of Maternal-Fetal Medicine, Department of Obstetrics and Gynecology, Sutter Health, California Pacific Medical Center, San Francisco, CA, USA; [b] Department of Surgery, University of California, Davis, Davis, CA, USA; [c] Department of Obstetrics and Gynecology, Oregon Health & Science University, Portland, OR, USA
* Corresponding author. 3700 California Street, Suite G330, San Francisco, CA 94118.
E-mail address: yvecheng@hotmail.com

Obstet Gynecol Clin N Am 44 (2017) 547–566
http://dx.doi.org/10.1016/j.ogc.2017.08.009
0889-8545/17/© 2017 Elsevier Inc. All rights reserved.

obgyn.theclinics.com

DEFINING NORMAL AND ABNORMAL LENGTH OF SECOND STAGE

The length of the second stage of labor is defined as the duration between complete cervical dilation and delivery of the fetus. Labor and delivery practice during the past half century have been based primarily on the work of Dr Emmanuel Friedman in the 1950s.[1,2] The American College of Obstetricians and Gynecologists (ACOG) Practice Bulletin No. 49 on Dystocia and Augmentation of Labor states that the mean durations of the second stage in nulliparous and multiparous women are 54 and 19 minutes, respectively,[3,4] and notes that the use of epidural analgesia increases these means by 25 minutes.[5] According to this ACOG Practice Bulletin, a prolonged second stage is defined as more than 2 hours without epidural or 3 hours with epidural analgesia in nulliparous women, and 1 hour without, or 2 hours with epidural analgesia for multiparous women.[3]

This definition of normal and abnormal length of the second stage is primarily based on Friedman's studies of 500 nulliparous[1] and 500 multiparous parturients,[2] using the 95th centile lengths of the second stage as the thresholds while incorporating expert opinions in attempt to prevent maternal and neonatal morbidity and mortality.[1-3,6,7] The additional hour allotted for labor with epidural anesthesia appears to be based on the mean effect of epidural.[8,9]

Recognizing that contemporary obstetric population and practice have evolved, a large, multicentered, prospective cohort study (Consortium of Safe Labor) was conducted between 2002 and 2008 to examine labor characteristics of women with spontaneous labor and normal neonatal outcomes in the United States.[10] This study included 43,810 nulliparous and 59,605 multiparous singleton deliveries at 36 weeks' gestation or greater in vertex presentation who reached second stage from 12 clinical centers with 19 hospitals.[10] In this study, the prevalence of prolonged second stage, as defined by the ACOG's guidelines,[3] occurred in 9.9% of nulliparous women with epidural and 13.9% of nulliparous women without epidural in labor.[11] For multiparous women, prolonged second stage was diagnosed in 3.1% with and 3.5% without an epidural in labor, respectively.[11] Such prevalence of prolonged second stage was similar to a large population-based study (n = 193,823) from Nova Scotia that spanned 19 years (1988–2006).[12] In this study, 14.8% of nulliparous and 3.2% of multiparous women were identified as having a second stage of labor longer than 3 hours, or 2 hours, respectively.[12] Furthermore, the annual incidence rates of prolonged second stage in nulliparous women increased from 10.2% to 16.6% during the study period.[12] These large studies demonstrate that the current definition of normal/abnormal second stage identifies a relatively high proportion (~15%) of the contemporary obstetric population as having a prolonged second stage. As such, it is of vital importance to ascertain the benefits and risks associated with the current definitions of normal and abnormal second stage and the management thereof.

FACTORS INFLUENCING LENGTH OF SECOND STAGE
Maternal and Obstetric Characteristics

Many clinical factors can influence the progress of the second stage of labor. These factors include maternal characteristics, such as age, parity, the size and shape of the pelvis, height and weight, uterine contractile forces, soft tissue resistance, expulsion effort, as well as presence of medical/obstetric conditions, including hypertensive disorders or pregestational/gestational diabetes mellitus. Fetal characteristics include birth weight, fetal occiput position/degree of flexion, and station at complete cervical dilation.[11,13-17] Interestingly, the duration of the second stage of labor in women who had induction of labor were similar to that of women who had spontaneous labor.[18]

Nevertheless, women with protracted first stage of labor (greater than the 95th centile, or 15.6 hours in this study) are more likely (16.3%) to also have a prolonged second stage of greater than the 95th centile in duration (2.9 hours) compared with women whose second stage was not protracted (4.5%, P<.001).[19]

Recent studies suggest that the progression of labor in modern obstetrics may have changed from the labor norms established by Friedman and data from the National Collaborative Perinatal Project (CPP) in the 1960s.[20,21] Zhang and colleagues[10] noted that the rate of cervical dilation in nulliparous women is substantially slower in the active phase and the descent of fetal head also can take longer during the second stage compared with "Friedman's labor curve."[1,2,11,22,23] According to the Consortium on Safe Labor, a large multicentered study of women in spontaneous, cervical dilation, particularly from 4 cm to 6 cm, is significantly slower for both nulliparous and multiparous women compared with that described by Friedman or the CPP cohort.[1,2,10,11,21,24] More specifically, the 95th centile threshold of duration was longer than 6 hours for cervical dilation to progress from 4 to 5 cm, and it was more than 3 hours for the cervix to progress from 5 to 6 cm.[10,21] The median length of the second stage of labor for women was also longer in comparison (nulliparous women with spontaneous delivery: median length 0.9 hour, 95th centile 3.1 hour).[10,11,21]

Although the precise reasons for observed variation in labor progression remain uncertain, differences in maternal characteristics and labor management have been postulated as potential contributors. Compared with women in the 1950s and 1960s, parturients today tend to delay childbearing, have increased maternal body mass index (BMI), and be of diverse racial/ethnic backgrounds; these factors have been associated with increased risk of labor dystocia and operative delivery, particularly during the first stage.[1,10,11,24–30] Besides changing maternal factors, management of labor has also evolved with time. The incidence of induction of labor is much higher today compared with decades prior.[31–33] Utilization of epidural analgesia during labor, and oxytocin augmentation of labor, is much more prevalent as part of labor management today,[11,34,35] and electronic fetal heart rate monitoring during labor and delivery is nearly universal.[36–38] In addition, there are substantially lower rates of forceps and vacuum-assisted vaginal deliveries.[39–42]

Impact of Epidural Analgesia: Maternal Effect

Epidural analgesia, nerve blockade via injection/infusion of local anesthetic/opioid analgesic agents into the lumbar epidural space, is widely used as a form of pain relief during labor and delivery. Although epidural analgesia offers better pain relief with higher satisfaction compared with other pharmacologic agents, it is also associated with higher likelihood of maternal hypotension (relative risk [RR] 18.23, 95% confidence interval [CI] 5.09–65.35), fever (RR 3.34, 95% CI 2.63–4.23), motor blockade (RR 31.67, 95% CI 4.33–231.51), and urinary retention (RR 17.05, 95% CI 4.82–60.39).[43–46]

Impact of Epidural Analgesia: Length of Labor

According to the Consortium on Safe Labor study, nulliparous women who had epidural analgesia in labor had a median duration of the second stage of 66 minutes, whereas those without epidural had a median second stage of 36 minutes (ie, median was 30 minutes longer second stage with epidural).[10] However, because the lengths of first and second stages of labor are not of normal distribution, examination of labor duration is more appropriately reported using the median and the 95th centile thresholds. Particularly, the 95th centile threshold customarily has been used to define an extreme of the labor distribution.[10,22,23,47–49] As such, the 95th centile duration of the second stage in nulliparous women with epidural was 3.6 hours and the 95th centile duration for those without epidural analgesia was 2.8 hours.[10] Thus, although the median length of the second stage among nulliparous women with and without epidural was 30 minutes different in duration, the 95th centile duration of the second stage was nearly 1 hour longer. For multiparous women, the 95th centile of the second stage ranged between 1.6 hours (for parity 2 or more) and 2.0 hours (for parity 1) with labor epidural analgesia, compared with 1.1 hours (for parity 2 or more) to 1.3 hours (for parity 1) in duration for those without epidural analgesia.[10] Similar associations between epidural and length of the second stage of labor at the median and the 95th centile thresholds have been observed in other large cohort studies of women who achieved vaginal delivery without adverse neonatal outcomes.[50,51]

Impact of Epidural Analgesia: Operative Interventions

Epidural analgesia, whether administered early or late in labor, does not appear to increase the risk of cesarean delivery compared with systemic opioid analgesia use.[34,52–56] A recent Cochrane systematic review of 9 randomized controlled trials including 15,752 women reports no difference in the duration of the second stage among women who had early versus late initiation of epidural analgesia in labor.[57] However, epidural analgesia has been implicated to affect labor progression, with increased need for oxytocin administration, longer second stage of labor, and higher risk of operative (forceps or vacuum-assisted) vaginal delivery,[34,43,58] although whether epidural truly increases the risk of operative vaginal delivery for dystocia remains debatable.[59–62] Despite high prevalence of epidural use for pain control in labor, its routine use, compared with on-request, can be associated with more operative interventions, adverse maternal effect (eg, hypotension, motor blockade) while not cost-effective. Thus, routine epidural analgesia administration is not encouraged; rather, women should make informed choices about labor analgesia.[63,64]

MANAGEMENT OF SECOND STAGE OF LABOR
Epidural Analgesia: Delayed Versus Immediate Pushing

For women who choose epidural analgesia for pain control during labor, the optimal management of the second stage remains debatable. Epidural analgesia along with concomitant sensory blockade can diminish a woman's urge to push in the second stage of labor.[65] Conventionally, parturients in the United States have been coached to begin pushing immediately upon complete cervical dilation in an effort to decrease the length of the second stage. This practice likely stemmed from the historic concerns that a prolonged second stage of labor was associated with peripartum asphyxia and fetal/neonatal death.[3,66,67] With better ability for and interpretation of intrapartum fetal monitoring,[68–70] some proposed that a longer second stage is not necessarily detrimental to the fetus in the presence of reassuring monitoring such that delayed pushing while allowing for passive descent of the fetal head can maximize the efficiency of maternal expulsive effort and may be a reasonable management option.[71–76]

One large multicenter, randomized controlled trial of "Pushing Early or Pushing Late with Epidural" (PEOPLE Study Group) compared 936 nulliparous women advised to wait for 2 hours or more after complete cervical dilation (delayed pushing or laboring down) before commencement of pushing to 926 nulliparous women who started pushing as soon as they reached the second stage.[77] The median durations of the second stage were 187 minutes (10th and 95th centile thresholds were 86 and 314 minutes, respectively) in the delayed pushing group versus 123 minutes (10th and 95th centile being 49 and 248 minutes, respectively) in the early pushing group.[77] Although women with delayed pushing had a shorter duration of pushing efforts (81.8 ± 61.2 minutes) compared with women with immediate pushing (117.9 ± 70.9 minutes), one-third of the entire study cohort had pushing effort of 2 to 3 hours, or 3 hours and longer.[77] There was no difference in the risk of cesarean delivery, but spontaneous vaginal delivery was more frequent among women who had delayed pushing compared with immediate pushing.[77] However, when examined by midpelvic or low/outlet procedures, it was only the midpelvic operative vaginal deliveries that were decreased by the process of laboring down. Furthermore, the rate of neonates with an abnormal umbilical artery gas, defined as a pH <7.1, was greater in the delayed pushing arm (4.5%) as compared with the immediate pushing arm (1.8%, $P<.05$).[77]

Other randomized controlled trials of nulliparous women with epidural analgesia compared immediate pushing with delayed pushing did not observe a difference in operative vaginal delivery nor risk of altered fecal continence or anal sphincter injury post delivery.[65,78]

However, a recent secondary analysis of a large cohort study consisted of 21,034 women, 18.4% (n = 3870) of whom had delayed pushing, and showed that delayed pushing was associated with higher risk of cesarean delivery (11.2% compared with 5.1% with immediate pushing, adjusted odds ratio [aOR] 1.86, 95% CI 1.63–2.21), higher risk of operative vaginal delivery (aOR 1.26, 95% CI 1.14–1.40), and maternal morbidity, including postpartum hemorrhage (aOR 1.43, 95% CI 1.05–1.95) and blood transfusion (aOR 1.51, 95% CI 1.04–2.17) with no differences in neonatal outcomes.[79] A meta-analysis of 12 randomized controlled trails that totaled 1,582 women with immediate and 1,531 delayed pushing showed that operative vaginal delivery rates were high in most studies but not significantly different between delayed (33.7%) and immediate pushing (37.4%, pooled RR 0.89, 95% CI 0.76–1.06).[80] Delayed pushing was associated with a longer second stage of labor (weighed mean difference 56.92 minutes, 95% CI 42.19–71.64) and shorter duration of active pushing (weighed mean difference −21.98 minutes, 95% CI −41.29 to −12.68) but few clinical differences in outcomes.[80] One prospective study did show that delayed pushing is associated with reduced maternal postpartum fatigue measured by the Modified Fatigue Symptom Checklist.[75]

Given debatable differences in outcomes associated with delayed versus immediate pushing among women opting for epidural analgesia in labor, management of the second stage may be guided by patient desire and provider preference as opposed to outcome driven. Nevertheless, nulliparity, maternal BMI greater than 25 kg/m^2, high fetal occiput station at complete cervical dilation, and start of the second stage during staffing shift change have been identified as independent factors associated with increased adoption of delayed pushing.[81] Interestingly, black race and second stage management during the night shift were associated with lower likelihood of delayed pushing.[81]

Epidural Analgesia: Discontinuation Late in Labor

For women with dense epidural analgesia who lack the urge to push, one management option that has been suggested is turning off the epidural to allow resumption of sensory and motor nerve function. A Cochrane systematic review identified 5 prospective, randomized trials (n = 462) that examined discontinuation of epidural analgesia late in labor and associated perinatal outcomes and reported no difference in mode of delivery or neonatal outcomes.[82] Although the second stage of labor was found to be slightly shorter, the proportion of women with inadequate pain relief increased dramatically (RR = 3.68 [1.99–6.80]).[82] Thus, halting epidural analgesia in the second stage does not appear to be an optimal management strategy. An alternative is to titrate the epidural dosing down to allow for greater motor capability while maintaining adequate analgesia.

Epidural Analgesia and Fetal Occiput Malposition

In addition to epidural analgesia potentially affecting maternal expulsive efforts and efficiency, some studies suggest that epidural analgesia may be associated with fetal head malposition (eg, occiput posterior or transverse position) at delivery, which may in turn contribute to higher rates of operative vaginal delivery and cesarean delivery.[83,84] One prospective study of 1,562 women evaluated changes in fetal position during labor using serial ultrasound examinations. This study reported that regardless of fetal head position early in labor, final fetal position is established close to delivery, and epidural is associated with higher likelihood of fetal occiput posterior position at delivery (12.9% with epidural vs 3.3% with no epidural, $P = .002$).[85] Interestingly, this study did not observe a higher incidence of occiput posterior position at the enrollment (23.4% vs 26.0%, with and without epidural, respectively; $P = .90$), thus suggesting that the association between epidural analgesia and fetal occiput malposition may be due to the absence of rotation during labor.[85] The use of epidural analgesia is associated with a higher rate of fetal occiput posterior position at delivery, which may in term contribute to higher rate of operative delivery.[84,85] This association was seen particularly if epidural analgesia was administered before engagement of the fetal head.[86,87] However, other investigators did not observe increase in the incidence of fetal occiput malposition at vaginal delivery associated with epidural analgesia use in labor.[88–90] Possible explanations for these contradicting study findings include differences in study design, definition of fetal occiput malposition, timing of assessment, variation in labor management style, and inability to determine the cause/effect relationship between epidural analgesia and malposition.[91]

MANAGEMENT OF PROLONGED SECOND STAGE OF LABOR

For women whose second stage of labor becomes prolonged, the ACOG Practice Bulletin on "Dystocia and Augmentation of Labor" advocates clinical assessment of the parturient, fetus, and uterine contractile forces and notes that intervention is not necessary solely based on passage of time.[3] As delayed pushing during the second stage can be a management option in women with labor epidural analgesia without urge to push, some also advocate the second stage of labor shall be delineated as 2 phases: a passive decent phase that allows for decent of fetal occiput without maternal exertion effort, and an active pushing phase of maternal expulsion effort.[92]

Length of Active Pushing During Second Stage and Associated Outcomes

To examine the association between the duration of active pushing during second stage of labor and associated outcomes, a secondary analysis of the PEOPLE trial that included 1862 nulliparous women was done. The investigators showed that relative to the first hour of pushing, the likelihood of spontaneous vaginal delivery of a newborn without signs of asphyxia decreases significantly with every passing hour: 1- to 2-hour aOR 0.4, 95% CI 0.3 to 0.6 for women who delivered in the 1- to 2-hour period of the second stage; aOR 0.1, 95% CI 0.09 to 0.2 for women who delivered in the 2- to 3-hour period; aOR 0.03, 95% CI 0.02 to 0.05 for women who delivered with a second stage duration of 3 hours or longer.[93] The investigators also observed increased risk of postpartum hemorrhage and intrapartum fever after 2 hours of active pushing.[93] Similar association between active pushing (but not passive decent) time and risk of postpartum hemorrhage was seen in a large prospective study of 3330 low-risk nulliparous women who achieved vaginal delivery: 1.2% for active second stage less than 10 minutes, 1.6% for 10–19 minutes, 2.1% for 20–29 minutes, 2.6% for 30–39 minutes, 4.5% for 40–49 minutes, and 14.3% for ≥50 minutes; aOR 10.5, 95% CI 28–40.3 for ≥50 minutes compared with less than 10 minutes.[94] Interestingly, a large population-based study from Sweden of 57,267 nulliparous women with term, singleton, vertex, live births delivered vaginally observed that the risk of postpartum hemorrhage increased with each passing hour of total second stage length as well as duration of pushing time.[95]

Given these findings, there appears to be a time threshold beyond which the probability of spontaneous vaginal delivery diminishes while risk of maternal morbidity increases such that it might not be reasonable to consider "stop pushing". However, a specific absolute maximum length of the second stage beyond which all women shall undergo operative delivery has not been established.

Timing of Operative Intervention and Associated Perinatal Outcomes

The question of "when to stop pushing" should balance the benefit of continuing pushing to achieve spontaneous vaginal delivery versus the potential need for operative intervention. One retrospective cohort study examined nulliparous women with singleton pregnancy at term who underwent operative vaginal delivery between 1 and 3 hours of the second stage compared with women who had vaginal delivery (by either spontaneous or operative vaginal delivery) at a later time. The investigators report that women who delivered later (>3 hours of the second stage) had a lower risk of third- or fourth-degree perineal laceration (aOR 0.63, 95% CI 0.51–0.77) without incurring increased risk of adverse neonatal outcome (neonatal cephalohematoma aOR 0.48, 95% CI 0.28–0.83; neonatal intensive care unit [NICU] admission aOR 0.70, 95% CI 0.49–0.99).[96]

Although the literature supports that a longer second stage of labor is associated with increased perinatal morbidity, such risk may not be entirely due to length of the second stage. Given that operative deliveries are more likely to occur due to passage of time, at least some of the morbidity with prolonged second stage may be due to such interventions. However, with close antepartum surveillance and continual labor progress, a prolonged second stage may not necessarily require operative intervention. As such, the Obstetric Care Consensus document on Safe Prevention of the Primary Cesarean Delivery, jointly developed by the ACOG and the Society for Maternal-Fetal Medicine (SMFM), recommends that at least 2 hours of pushing in multiparous women, and at least 3 hours of pushing in nulliparous women (if maternal and fetal conditions permit) be allowed before the diagnosis of labor arrest in the second stage.[97] Additional time to these thresholds should be allowed with an epidural or fetal malposition.

PERINATAL OUTCOMES ASSOCIATED WITH LENGTH OF SECOND STAGE

Defining appropriate duration of the second stage of labor is challenging because management involves careful consideration of maternal and neonatal outcomes, which are often competing. Current available data suggest that as the duration of the second stage of labor increases, so does the likelihood of operative interventions and maternal morbidity. Data on neonatal outcome are less clear.

Length of Second Stage and Associated Maternal Outcomes

The inverse relationship of length of the second stage and odds of spontaneous vaginal delivery has been well established. In examining nulliparous women (n = 1862) with labor epidural analgesia (secondary analysis of the PEOPLE study), the probably of spontaneous vagina delivery without neonatal asphyxia was ~50% during the first hour of active pushing; this probability decreases to ~20% after 2 hours of active pushing and further decreases to 10% after 3 hours or more of active pushing.[93] A similar association was seen in another secondary analysis of multicentered, large cohort study of nulliparous reached the second stage (n = 4126).[98] In this analysis, the frequency of spontaneous vaginal delivery decreased with length of the second stage: 85% with the second stage less than 1 hour, 78% with the second stage 1 to 2 hours, 59% with the second stage 2 to 3 hours, 27% with the second stage 3 to 4 hours, and 25% with the second stage 4 to 5 hours, and 9% when the second stage lasted 5 hours or longer.[98] In addition, compared with cesarean deliveries performed during the first stage, cesarean delivery during the second stage is associated with statistically significantly longer operative time, and intraoperative complications such as uterine atony, a T or J uterine incision extension, and incidental cystotomy; the composite maternal morbidity was 19.6% for cesarean deliveries in the first stage and 21.7% in the second stage (aOR 1.13; 95% CI 1.02–1.26).[99]

Besides decreasing likelihood of spontaneous vaginal delivery with increasing length of the second stage, a longer second stage is associated with increased risk of maternal morbidity, including puerperal infection, third- and fourth-degree perineal lacerations, and postpartum hemorrhage as well as operative vaginal delivery and episiotomy (**Table 1**).[11,12,92–95,98,100–102] Although the association between length of labor and maternal morbidity is consistent in the existing literature, it remains debatable whether such association is causal (ie, whether a long labor results in chorioamnionitis, or that chorioamnionitis causes ineffective uterine contractions that lead to prolonged second stage). Finally, clinicians are more likely to offer operative intervention in the presence of a longer second stage, and operative intervention is associated with increased risk of perineal lacerations and postpartum hemorrhage. Because the extent to which the length of the second stage contributes to maternal morbidity, and vice versa, remains unclear, the goal of managing second stage of labor shall be to maximize the probability of vaginal delivery while minimizing the risks of perinatal morbidity.[103]

Length of Second Stage and Associated Neonatal Outcome: Nulliparous Women

The second stage of labor is historically considered to be a time during which the fetus would be at high risk of asphyxia. With widespread availability and utilization of fetal monitoring in labor, several large cohort studies suggest that the length of the second stage is not associated with adverse neonatal outcome in nulliparous women. In multiple large cohort studies of nulliparous women who reached the second stage of labor, length of the second stage was not associated with short-term undesirable neonatal measures, such as low 5-minute Apgar score less than 7 or umbilical cord arterial pH <7.0,[93,100,101,104,105] although the data on NICU admission and risk of birth trauma remained mixed, and some studies report adverse neonatal outcome associated with length of the second stage (**Table 2**).[12,51,98,102,106]

A secondary analysis of data from the Consortium on Safe Labor was able to examine neonatal outcomes associated with a prolonged second stage of labor, compared with second stage of labor within the ACOG guidelines,[3] with stratification by parity and status of epidural analgesia use in labor.[102] For nulliparous women with

Table 1
Maternal morbidity associated with the length of the second stage

Author	Study Design	Subjects	Summary of Finding: aOR and 95% CI
Allen et al,[12] 2009	Population-based retrospective cohort study (1988–2006)	N = 121,517	Nulliparous women with >3 h of second stage compared with <2 h: Increase in risk of obstetric trauma (aOR 1.84 [1.65–2.06]), postpartum hemorrhage (aOR 1.53 [1.37–1.72]), puerperal febrile morbidity (aOR 1.63 [1.39–1.92])
Le Ray et al,[93] 2009	Secondary analysis of multicentered randomized controlled study (1994–1996)	N = 1863	Nulliparous women >3 h pushing duration compared with <1 h: Increase in risk of postpartum hemorrhage (aOR 2.5 [1.5–4.1]) and intrapartum fever (aOR 2.7 [1.3–5.5])
Looft et al,[95] 2017	Population-based cohort study (2008–2014)	N = 57,267	Each additional hour of second stage: compared with a second stage <1h, the adjusted RR for PPH were for 1 to <2 h, RR 1.10, 95% CI 1.07–1.14; for 2 to <3 h, RR 1.15 (95% CI 1.10–1.20); for 3 to <4 h, RR 1.28 (95% CI 1.22–1.33); and for ≥4 h, RR 1.40 (95% CI 1.33–1.46) RR of PPH also increased with pushing time >30 min: for 30–44 min, RR 1.08 (95% CI 104–1.12); for 45–59 min, RR 1.11 (95% CI 1.06–1.16); for >60 min, RR 1.20 (95% CI 1.15–1.25)
Cheng et al,[96] 2011	Single-institution retrospective cohort study (1976–2001)	N = 15,759	Nulliparous women with >3 h of second stage compared with <3 h: Increased risk of postpartum hemorrhage (aOR 1.48 [1.24–1.78]), and chorioamnionitis (aOR 2.14 [1.80–2.57])

(continued on next page)

Table 1
(continued)

Author	Study Design	Subjects	Summary of Finding: aOR and 95% CI
Rouse et al,[98] 2009	Secondary analysis of multicentered trial	N = 4126	Each additional hour of second stage in nulliparous women: Increased risk of chorioamnionitis (aOR 1.60 [1.40–1.83]), third- or fourth-degree perineal laceration (aOR 1.44 [1.29–1.60]), and uterine atony (aOR 1.31 [1.14–1.51])
Saunders et al,[100] 1992	Multicentered retrospective cohort study (1988)	N = 25,069	Increased risk of postpartum hemorrhage and infection
Myles & Santolaya,[101] 2003	Single-institution retrospective cohort study (1996–1999)	N = 6791	Increased risk of perineal trauma, episiotomy usage, chorioamnionitis, and postpartum hemorrhage
Laughon et al,[102] 2014	Multicentered cohort study (2002–2008)	N = 103,415	Prolonged second stage compared with no prolonged second stage by ACOG criteria[3]: Increased risk of endometritis (aOR 3.52 [2.44–5.06]), postpartum hemorrhage (aOR 1.50 [1.27–1.78]), chorioamnionitis (aOR 3.01 [2.65–3.43]), and 3rd/4th degree perineal laceration (aOR 1.80 [1.58–2.05]) for nulliparous women with epidural; increased risk of postpartum hemorrhage (aOR 1.50 [1.07–2.10]), chorioamnionitis (aOR 4.78 [3.46–6.61]), episiotomy (aOR1.44 [1.21–1.70]), and 3rd/4th degree perineal laceration (aOR 3.85 [2.65–5.60]) for multiparous women with epidural

Abbreviation: PPH, postpartum hemorrhage.

Table 2
Neonatal outcomes associated with the length of the second stage

Author	Study Design	Subjects	Summary of Finding: aOR and 95% CI
Length of second stage not associated with neonatal morbidity			
Le Ray et al,[93] 2009	Secondary analysis of multicentered randomized controlled study (1994–1996)	N = 1863	Nulliparous women >3 h pushing duration compared with <1 h: No increased risk of adverse neonatal outcome: 5-min Apgar <7 (aOR 0.7 [0.1–1.1]), arterial pH <7.10 (aOR 0.2 [0.1–1.1]), neonatal trauma (aOR 1.7 [0.9–3.3]), admission to NICU (aOR 1.5 [0.7–3.3])
Saunders et al,[100] 1992	Multicentered retrospective cohort study (1988)	N = 25,069	No increased risk of adverse neonatal outcome
Myles & Santolaya,[101] 2003	Single-institution, retrospective cohort study (1996–1999)	N = 6791	No differences in neonatal morbidity
Janni et al,[104] 2002	Single-institution, retrospective cohort study (1999–2000)	N = 1457	Prolonged second stage >2 h not associated with low 5-min Apgar scores, umbilical artery pH <7.0, NICU admission
Cheng et al,[105] 2004	Single-institution, retrospective cohort study (1976–2001)	N = 15,759	Nulliparous women with >3 h of second stage compared with <3 h: No increased risk of adverse neonatal outcome: 5-min Apgar <7 (aOR 0.73 [0.48–1.11]), umbilical artery pH <7.0 (aOR 1.21 [0.45–3.29]), base excess <−12 (aOR 0.61 [0.32–1.16]), NICU admission (aOR 1.07 [0.72–1.58])
Length of second stage associated with neonatal morbidity			
Allen et al,[12] 2009	Cohort study (1988–2006)	N = 121,517	Nulliparous women with >3 h of second stage compared with <2 h: increased risk of 5-min Apgar score <7 (aOR 1.35 [1.04–1.77]), birth depression (delay in initiating and maintaining respiration after birth and requiring resuscitation by oxygen mask or endotracheal tube for at least 3 min; aOR 1.59 [1.29–1.97]), and admission to the NICU (aOR 1.94 [1.74–2.16])

(continued on next page)

Table 2
(continued)

Author	Study Design	Subjects	Summary of Finding: aOR and 95% CI
Cheng et al,[50] 2004	Single-institution retrospective cohort study (1976–2008)	N = 42,268	Prolonged second stage compared with no prolonged second stage by ACOG definition[3]: Increased risk of birth trauma (composite variable for cephalohematoma, head laceration, clavicular fracture, skull fracture, facial nerve palsy, and brachial plexus palsy; aOR 1.58 [1.13–2.22])
Rouse et al,[98] 2009	Secondary analysis of multicentered trial	N = 4126	Each additional hour of second stage in nulliparous women: Increased risk brachial plexus injury (aOR 1.78 [1.08–2.78])
Laughon et al,[102] 2014	Multicentered cohort study (2002–2008)	N = 103,415	Prolonged second stage compared with no prolonged second stage by ACOG criteria[3]: Increase in risk of neonatal sepsis in nulliparous women (with epidural aOR 2.08 [1.60–2.70] and without epidural aOR 2.34 [1.28–4.27]), asphyxia in nulliparous with epidural (aOR 2.39 [1.22–4.66]), and perinatal mortality without epidural (aOR 5.92 [1.43–24.51] for nulliparous and aOR 6.34 [1.32–30.34] for multiparous women)
Sandstrom et al,[106] 2017	Population-based cohort study (2008–2013)	N = 42,539	Prolonged second stage (<1 h vs ≥4 h) associated with increased RR of birth asphyxia (RR 2.46, 95% CI 1.66–3.66), NICU admission (RR 1.80, 95% CI 1.58–2.04) Pushing duration (<15 min vs ≥60 min) associated with increased risk of academia (RR 2.55, 95% CI 1.51–4.30)

epidural, neonatal morbidity is associated with a prolonged second stage compared with length of the second stage within guidelines. Such morbidity included higher odds of 5-minute Apgar score less than 4 (0.5% vs 0.2%; aOR 2.71, 95% CI 1.49–4.93), NICU admission (8.2% vs 5.9%; aOR 1.39, 95% CI 1.20–1.60), sepsis (2.6% vs 1.2%; aOR 2.08, 95% CI 1.60–2.70), and asphyxia (0.3% vs 0.1%; aOR 2.39, 95% CI 1.22–4.66). For nulliparous women without epidural but with a prolonged second stage, their neonates had higher odds of sepsis (1.8% vs 1.1%; aOR 2.34, 95% CI 1.28–4.27) as well as a near 6-fold increase in risk of perinatal mortality (0.18% vs 0.04%; aOR 5.92, 95% CI 1.43–24.51).[102] Although the absolute incidence rate of asphyxia and perinatal mortality were low (<0.5%), these detrimental outcomes can, and likely will, have profound clinical and psychological impact on both the patient/family and clinicians.

Length of Active Pushing and Associated Neonatal Outcome

Although most studies on the length of the second stage did not distinguish the duration of delayed pushing/passive descent versus the duration of active pushing, a secondary analysis of nulliparous women with epidural analgesia observed that neonatal outcomes of women who pushed for greater than 3 hours were not statistically significantly different from those with less than 1 hour of active pushing: Apgar less than 7 at 5 minutes (1.6% vs 0.8%; aOR 0.7, 95% CI 0.1–3.5), umbilical cord arterial pH ≤7.10 (1.4% vs 3.6%; aOR 0.2, 95% CI 0.1–1.1), neonatal trauma (12.3% vs 5.4%; aOR 1.7, 95% CI 0.9–3.3), and NICU admission (8.6% vs 3.5%; aOR 1.5, 95% CI 0.7–3.3).[93] However, a large population-based study from Sweden did observe a pushing time of ≥60 minutes, compared with less than 15 minutes, was associated with increased risk of academia: 0.57% for less than 15 minutes pushing vs 1.69% for ≥60 minutes of pushing (RR 2.55, 95% CI 1.51–4.30).[106]

Length of Second Stage and Associated Neonatal Outcome: Multiparous Women

Few studies exist regarding neonatal outcomes associated with the length of the second stage in multiparous women. A prolonged second stage in multiparous women with epidural analgesia is associated with a higher risk of 5-minute Apgar less than 4 (0.4% vs 0.2%; aOR 2.52, 95% CI 1.01–6.30) and NICU admission (6.2% vs 4.1%; aOR 1.57, 95% CI 1.22–2.03).[102] For those with a prolonged second stage without epidural analgesia, their neonates are more likely to experience shoulder dystocia (2.2% vs 1.7%; aOR 1.78, 95% CI 1.02–3.09), need respiratory resuscitation with continuous positive airway pressure or more (0.6% vs 0.4%; aOR 2.53, 95% CI 1.06–6.05), and are at higher risk of perinatal death compared with those without a prolonged second stage (0.21% and 0.03%; aOR 6.34, 95% CI 1.32–30.34).[102] Similarly, 2 additional large cohort studies also showed neonates born to multiparous women with a prolonged second stage, particularly 3 hours or longer, are more likely to have a 5-minute Apgar less than 7 (aOR 2.24, 95% CI 1.25–4.00), birth depression (aOR 1.68; 95% CI 1.05–2.70), NICU admission (aOR 1.55; 95% CI 1.20–2.00), and longer hospital stay (aOR 1.67; 95% CI 1.11–2.51) compared with those born without a prolonged second stage.[12,107]

Although multiparous women are expected to have a shorter second stage of labor, when a prolonged second stage does occur in multiparous women, it may be a manifestation of true cephalopelvic disproportion or fetal head malposition. Given the association of a prolonged second stage and adverse neonatal outcome and potential perinatal death, close fetal surveillance with thoughtful balance of risks and benefits for both the mother and the neonate is essential to achieve optimal obstetric and perinatal outcome. In addition, the observation that perinatal mortality was more frequent in both nulliparous and multiparous women with a prolonged second stage without epidural analgesia in labor warrants further investigation because the precise cause for this association remains unknown. Perhaps, a prolonged second stage in the presence of epidural analgesia is less ominous than a protracted labor, resulting in prolonged second stage from other pathophysiology.

SUMMARY

Although the ACOG's Practice Bulletin on labor historically defined a prolonged second stage of labor in nulliparous women as a lack of progress for 2 hours without or 3 hours with epidural analgesia, and for multiparous, 1 hour without or 2 hours with epidural, in 2000,[3] more recently, the *Eunice Kennedy Shriver* National Institute of Child Health and Human Development, the SMFM, and the ACOG convened a joint workshop to strategize about the prevention of the first cesarean delivery.[108] This document suggested that second stage arrest be defined as no progress in descent or rotation for 3 hours or more in nulliparous women without epidural and 4 hours or more for nulliparous women with epidural analgesia; similarly, for multiparous women, 2 hours or more without and 3 hours or more with epidural analgesia.[108] Furthermore, the first Obstetric Care Consensus Document, developed jointly by ACOG and the SMFM, suggests that 2 hours of pushing time for multiparous, 3 hours of pushing for nulliparous women, be permitted (if fetal/maternal evaluation continues to be reassuring) before diagnosing arrest of labor in the second stage.[97] Both documents stress that progress in the second stage involves descent and rotation of the fetal head as the fetus traverses the maternal pelvis. Thus, protracted labor in itself should not be the sole indication for operative intervention if progress is being made in the presence of reassuring maternal and fetal status. Further research into length and management of the second stage is needed to produce the evidence to guide our practice.

REFERENCES

1. Friedman EA. Primigravid labor; a graphicostatistical analysis. Obstet Gynecol 1955;6:567–89.
2. Friedman EA. Labor in multiparas; a graphicostatistical analysis. Obstet Gynecol 1956;8:691–703.
3. American College of Obstetrics and Gynecology Committee on Practice Bulletins-Obstetrics. ACOG Practice Bulletin number 49, December 2003: dystocia and augmentation of labor. Obstet Gynecol 2003;102:1445–54.
4. Kilpatrick SJ, Laros RK Jr. Characteristics of normal labor. Obstet Gynecol 1989; 74:85–7.
5. Zhang J, Yancey MK, Klebanoff MA, et al. Does epidural analgesia prolong labor and increase risk of cesarean delivery? A natural experiment. Am J Obstet Gynecol 2001;185:128–34.
6. Hellman LM, Prystowsky H. The duration of the second stage of labor. Am J Obstet Gynecol 1952;63:1223–33.
7. Hamilton G. On the proper management of tedious labors. Br Foreign Med Chir Rev 1971;48:449.
8. Albers LL. The duration of labor in healthy women. J Perinatol 1999;19:1114–9.
9. Albers LL, Schiff M, Gorwoda JG. The length of active labor in normal pregnancies. Obstet Gynecol 1996;87:355–9.
10. Zhang J, Landy HJ, Branch DW, et al, Consortium on Safe Labor. Contemporary patterns of spontaneous labor with normal neonatal outcomes. Obstet Gynecol 2010;116:1281–7.

11. Laughon SK, Branch DW, Beaver J, et al. Changes in labor patterns over 50 years. Am J Obstet Gynecol 2012;206:419.e1-9.

12. Allen VM, Baskett TF, O'Connell CM, et al. Maternal and perinatal outcomes with increasing duration of the second stage of labor. Obstet Gynecol 2009;113:1248–58.

13. Sizer AR, Evans J, Bailey SM, et al. A second-stage partogram. Obstet Gynecol 2000;96:678–83.

14. Senécal J, Xiong X, Faser WD, Pushing Early or Pushing Late with Epidural study Group. Effect of fetal position on second-stage duration and labor outcome. Obstet Gynecol 2005;105:763–72.

15. Zaki MN, Hibbard JU, Kominiarek MA. Contemporary labor patterns and maternal age. Obstet Gynecol 2013;122:1018–24.

16. Piper JM, Bolling DR, Newton ER. The second stage of labor: factors influencing duration. Am J Obstet Gynecol 1991;165:97609.

17. Feinstein U, Sheiner E, Levy A, et al. Risk factors for arrest of descent during the second stage of labor. Int J Gynaecol Obstet 2002;77:7–14.

18. Janakiraman V, Ecker J, Kaimal AJ. Comparing the second stage in inducted and spontaneous labor. Obstet Gynecol 2010;116:606–11.

19. Nelson DB, McIntire DD, Leveno KJ. Relationship of the length of the first stage of labor to the length of the second stage. Obstet Gynecol 2013;122:27–32.

20. Friedman EA, Sachtleben MR. Station of the presenting part. I. Pattern of descent. Am J Obstet Gynecol 1965;93:552–9.

21. Zhang J, Troendle JF, Yancey MK. Reassessing the labor curve in nulliparous women. Am J Obstet Gynecol 2002;187:824–8.

22. Friedman E. The graphic analysis of labor. Am J Obstet Gynecol 1954;68:1568–75.

23. Zhang J, Troendle J, Mikolajczyk R, et al. The natural history of the normal first stage of labor. Obstet Gynecol 2010;115:705–10.

24. Kominiarek MA, Vanveldhuisen P, Hibbard J, et al, Consortium on Safe Labor. The maternal body mass index: a strong association with delivery route. Am J Obstet Gynecol 2010;203:264.e1-7.

25. Greenberg MB, Cheng YW, Sullivan M, et al. Does length of labor vary by maternal age? Am J Obstet Gynecol 2007;197:428.e1-7.

26. Greenberg MB, Cheng YW, Hopkins LM, et al. Are there ethnic differences in the length of labor? Am J Obstet Gynecol 2006;195:743–8.

27. Ecker JL, Chen KT, Cohen AP, et al. Increased risk of cesarean delivery with advancing maternal age: indications and associated factors in nulliparous women. Am J Obstet Gynecol 2001;185:883–7.

28. Traecy A, Robsn M, O'Herlihy C. Dystocia increases with advancing maternal age. Am J Obstet Gynecol 2006;195:760–3.

29. Hilliard AM, Chauhan SP, Zhao Y, et al. Effect of obesity on length of labor in nulliparous women. Am J Perinatol 2012;29:127–32.

30. Kawakita T, Reddy UM, Landy HJ, et al. Indications for primary cesarean delivery relative to body mass index. Am J Obstet Gynecol 2016;215:515.e1-9.

31. Bonsack CF, Lathrop A, Blackburn M. Induction of labor: update and review. J Midwifery Womens Health 2014;59:606–15.

32. Dojl M, Vanky E, Heimstad R. Changes in induction methods have not influenced cesarean section rates among women with induced labor. Acta Obstet Gynecol Scand 2016;95:112–5.

33. Baud D, Rouiller S, Hohlfeld P, et al. Adverse obstetrical and neonatal outcomes in elective and medically indicated inductions of labor at term. J Matern Fetal Neonatal Med 2013;26:1595–601.

34. Grant E, Tao W, Craig M, et al. Neuroaxial analgesia effects on labour progression: facts, fallacies, uncertainties and the future. BJOG 2015;122(3):288–93 [Epub ahead of print].

35. Martin JA, Hamilton BE, Ventura SJ, et al. Division of vital statistics. Births: final data for 2012. Natl Vital Stat Rep 2013;62:1–69.

36. Saldana LR, Schulman H, Yang WH. Electronic fetal monitoring during labor. Obstet Gynecol 1976;47:706–10.

37. Westgren M, Ingemarsson E, Ingemarsson I, et al. Intrapartum electronic fetal monitoring in low-risk pregnancies. Obstet Gynecol 1980;56:301–4.

38. Mueller-Heubach E, MacDonald HM, Joret D, et al. Effects of electronic fetal monitoring on perinatal outcome and obstetric practices. Am J Obstet Gynecol 1980;137:758–63.

39. Hirshberg A, Srinivas SK. Role of operative vaginal deliveries in prevention of cesarean deliveries. Clin Obstet Gynecol 2015;58:256–62.

40. Fitzwater JL, Owen J, Ankumah NA, et al. Nulliparous women in the second stage of labor: changes in delivery outcomes between two cohorts from 2000 and 2011. Obstet Gynecol 2015;126:81–6.

41. Ebulue V, Vadalkar J, Cely S, et al. Fear of failure: are we doing too many trials of instrumental delivery in theatre? Acta Obstet Gynecol Scand 2008;87:1234–8.

42. Cheong YC, Abdulahi H, Lashen H, et al. Can formal education and training improve the outcome of instrumental delivery? Eur J Obstet Gynecol Reprod Biol 2004;113:139–44.

43. Anim-Somuah M, Smyth RM, Jones L. Epidural versus non-epidural or no analgesia in labour. Cochrane Database Syst Rev 2011;(12):CD000331.

44. Collis RE, Davies DW, Aveling W. Randomized comparison of combined spinal-epidural and standard epidural analgesia in labour. Lancet 1995;345:1413–6.

45. Mayberry LJ, Clemmens D, De A. Epidural analgesia side effects, co-interventions, and care of women during childbirth: a systematic review. Am J Obstet Gynecol 2002;186:S81–93.

46. Yancey MK, Zhang J, Schwarz J, et al. Labor epidural analgesia and intrapartum maternal hyperthermia. Obstet Gynecol 2001;98:763–70.

47. Vahratian A, Zhang J, Troendle JF, et al. Maternal prepregnancy overweight and obesity and the pattern of labor progression in term nulliparous women. Obstet Gynecol 2004;104:943–51.

48. Graseck AS, Odibo AO, Tuuli M, et al. Normal first stage of labor in women undergoing trial of labor after cesarean delivery. Obstet Gynecol 2012;119:732–6.

49. Normal SM, Tuuli MG, Odibo AO, et al. The effects of obesity on the first stage of labor. Obstet Gynecol 2012;120:130–5.

50. Cheng YW, Shaffer BL, Nicholson JM, et al. Second stage of labor and epidural use: a larger effect than previously suggested. Obstet Gynecol 2004;123:527–35.

51. Hung TH, Chen SF, Lo LM, et al. Contemporary second stage labor patterns in Taiwanese women with normal neonatal outcomes. Taiwan J Obstet Gynecol 2015;54:416–20.

52. Wong CA, McCarthy RJ, Sullivan JT, et al. Early compared with late neuraxial analgesia in nulliparous labor induction: a randomize controlled trial. Obstet Gynecol 2009;113:1066–74.

53. Wong CA, Scavone BM, Peaceman AM, et al. The risk of cesarean delivery with neuraxial analgesia given early versus late in labor. N Engl J Med 2005;352: 655–65.
54. Wang F, Shen X, Gua X, et al, Labor Analgesia Examining Group. Epidural analgesia in the latent phase of labor and the risk of cesarean delivery: a five-year randomized controlled trial. Anesthesiology 2009;111:871–80.
55. Ohel G, Gonen R, Vaida S, et al. Early versus late initiation of epidural analgesia in labor: does it increase the risk of cesarean section? A randomized trial. Am J Obstet Gynecol 2006;194:600–5.
56. Leighton BL, Halpern SH. The effects of epidural analgesia on labor, maternal, and neonatal outcomes: a systematic review. Am J Obstet Gynecol 2002;186: S69–77.
57. Sng BL, Leong WL, Zeng Y, et al. Early versus late initiation of epidural analgesia for labour. Cochrane Database Syst Rev 2014;(10):CD007328.
58. Dickinson JE, Paech MJ, McDonald SJ, et al. The impact of intrapartum analgesia on labour and delivery outcomes in nulliparous women. Aust N Z J Obstet Gynaecol 2002;42:59–66.
59. Chestnut DH, Vincent RD Jr, McGarth JM, et al. Does early administration of epidural analgesia affect obstetric outcome in nulliparous women who are receiving intravenous oxytocin? Anesthesiology 1994;80:1193–200.
60. Yancey MK, Pierce B, Schweitzer D, et al. Observations on labor epidural analgesia and operative delivery rates. Am J Obstet Gynecol 1999;180:353–9.
61. Impey L, MacQuillan K, Robason M. Epidural analgesia need not increase operative delivery rates. Am J Obstet Gynecol 2000;182:358–63.
62. Halpern SH, Leighton BL, Ohlsson A, et al. Effect of epidural vs parenteral opioid analgesia on the progress of labor: a meta-analysis. JAMA 1998;280: 2105–10.
63. Wassen MM, Smits LJ, Scheepers HC, et al. Routine labour epidural analgesia versus labour analgesia on request: a randomized non-inferiority trial. BJOG 2015;112:344–50.
64. Bonouvrie K, van den Bosch A, Roumen FJ, et al. Epidural analgesia during labour, routinely or on request: a cost-effectiveness analysis. Eur J Obstet Gynecol Reprod Biol 2016;207:23–31.
65. Plunkett BA, Lin A, Wong CA, et al. Management of the second stage of labor in nulliparas with continuous epidural analgesia. Obstet Gynecol 2003;102: 109–14.
66. Friedman EA, Sachtleben MR. Station of the fetal presenting part. VI. Arrest of descent in nulliparas. Am J Obstet Gynecol 1976;47:129–36.
67. Clark SL, Hamilton EF, Garite TJ, et al. The limits of electronic fetal heart rate monitoring in the prevention of neonatal metabolic academia. Am J Obstet Gynecol 2017;216:163.e1-6.
68. American College of Obstetricians and Gynecologists. ACOG Practice Bulletin. Clinical Management Guidelines for Obstetrician-Gynecologists, Number 70, December 2005 (Replaces Practice Bulletin Number 62, May 2005). Intrapartum fetal heart rate monitoring. Obstet Gynecol 2005;106:1453–60.
69. Santo S, Ayres-de-Campos D, Costa-Santos C, et al. Agreement and accuracy using the FIGO, ACOG, NICE cardiotocography interpretation guidelines. Acta Obstet Gynecol Scand 2017;96:166–75.
70. Triebwasser JE, Colvin R, Macones GA, et al. Nonreassuring fetal status in the second stage of labor: fetal monitoring features and association with neonatal outcomes. Am J Perinatol 2016;33:665–70.

71. Maresh M, Choong KH, Beard RW. Delayed pushing with lumbar epidural analgesia in labour. Br J Obstet Gynaecol 1983;90:623–7.
72. Piquard F, Schaefer A, Hsiung R, et al. Are there two biological parts in the second stage of labor? Acta Obstet Gynecol Scand 1989;68:713–8.
73. Kopas ML. A review of evidence-based practices for management of the second stage of labor. J Midwifery Womens Health 2014;59:264–76.
74. Brancato RM, Church S, Stone PW. A meta-analysis of passive descent versus immediate pushing in nulliparous women with epidural analgesia in the second stage of labor. J Obstet Gynecol Neonatal Nurs 2008;37:4–12.
75. Lai ML, Lin KC, Li HY, et al. Effects of delayed pushing during the second stage of labor on postpartum fatigue and birth outcomes in nulliparous women. J Nurs Res 2009;17:62–72.
76. Hansen SL, Clark SL, Foster JC. Active pushing versus passive fetal descent in the second stage of labor: a randomized controlled trial. Obstet Gynecol 2002; 99:29–34.
77. Fraser WD, Marcoux S, Krauss I, et al. Multicenter, randomized, controlled trial of delayed pushing for nulliparous women in the second stage of labor with continuous epidural analgesia. The PEOPLE (Pushing Early or Pushing Late with Epidural) Study Group. Am J Obstet Gynecol 2000;182:1165–72.
78. Fizpatrick M, Harkin R, McQuillan K, et al. A randomised clinical trial comparing the effects of delayed versus immediate pushing with epidural analgesia on mode of delivery and faecal continence. BJOG 2002;109:1359–65.
79. Yee LM, Sandoval G, Bailit J, et al. Eunice Kennedy Shriver National Institute of Child Health and Human Development (NICHD) Maternal-Fetal Medicine Units (MFMU) Network. Maternal and neonatal outcomes with early compared with delayed pushing among nulliparous women. Obstet Gynecol 2016;128: 1039–47.
80. Tuuli MG, Frey HA, Odibo AO, et al. Immediate compared with delayed pushing in the second stage of labor: a systematic review and meta-analysis. Obstet Gynecol 2012;120:660–8.
81. Frey HA, Tuuli MG, Odibo AO, et al. Medical and nonmedical factors influencing utilization of delayed pushing in the second stage. Am J Perinatol 2013;30: 595–600.
82. Torvaldsen S, Roberts CL, Bell JC, et al. Discontinuation of epidural analgesia late in labour for reducing the adverse delivery outcomes associated with epidural analgesia. Cochrane Database Syst Rev 2004;(4):CD004457.
83. Sizer AR, Nirmal DM. Occipitoposterior position: associated factors and obstetric outcomes in nulliparas. Obstet Gynecol 2000;96:749–52.
84. Ponkey SE, Cohen AP, Heffner LJ, et al. Persistent fetal occiput posterior position: obstetric outcomes. Obstet Gynecol 2003;101:915–20.
85. Lieberman E, Davidson K, Lee-Parritz A, et al. Changes in fetal position during labor and their association with epidural analgesia. Obstet Gynecol 2005;105: 974–82.
86. Robinson CA, Macones GA, Roth NW, et al. Does station of the fetal head at epidural placement affect the position of the fetal vertex at delivery? Am J Obstet Gynecol 1996;175:991–4.
87. Le Ray C, Carayol M, Jaquemin S, et al. Is epidural analgesia a risk factor for occiput posterior or transverse position during labor? Eur J Obstet Gynecol Reprod Biol 2005;123:22–6.
88. Yancy MK, Zhang J, Schweitzer DL, et al. Epidural analgesia and fetal head malposition at vaginal delivery. Obstet Gynecol 2001;97:608–12.

89. Gardberg M, Laakkonen E, Salevaara M. Intrapartum sonography and persistent occiput posterior position: a study of 408 deliveries. Obstet Gynecol 1998;91:746–9.

90. Fitzpatrick M, McQuillan K, O'Herlihy C. Influence of persistent occiput posterior position on delivery outcome. Obstet Gynecol 2001;98:1027–31.

91. Lieberman E, O'Donoghue C. Unintended effects of epidural analgesia during labor: a systematic review. Am J Obstet Gynecol 2000;186(Suppl):S31–68.

92. Roberts JE. The "push" for evidence: management of the second stage. J Midwifery Womens Health 2002;47:2–15.

93. Le Ray C, Audibert F, Goffinet F, et al. When to stop pushing: effects of duration of second-stage expulsion efforts on maternal and neonatal outcomes in nulliparous women with epidural analgesia. Am J Obstet Gynecol 2009;201:361.e1-7.

94. Le Ray C, Fraser W, Rozenberg P, et al, PREMODA Study Group. Duration of passive and active phases of the second stage of labour and risk of severe postpartum haemorrhage in low-risk nulliparous women. Eur J Obstet Gynecol Reprod Biol 2011;158:167–72.

95. Looft E, Simic M, Ahlberg M, et al. Duration of second stage labour at term and pushing time: risk factors for postpartum haemorrhage. Paediatr Perinat Epidemiol 2017;31:126–33.

96. Cheng YW, Shaffer BL, Bianco K, et al. Timing of operative vaginal delivery and associated perinatal outcomes in nulliparous women. J Matern Fetal Neonatal Med 2011;24:692–7.

97. Caughey AB, Cahill AG, Guise JM, et al. ACOG/SMFM Obstetric Care Consensus. Safe prevention of the primary cesarean delivery. Obstet Gynecol 2014;123:693–711.

98. Rouse DJ, Weiner SJ, Bloom SL, et al, for the Eunice Kennedy Shriver National Institute of Child Health and Human Development Maternal-Fetal Medicine Units Network. Second-stage labor duration in nulliparous women: relationship to maternal and perinatal outcomes. Am J Obstet Gynecol 2009;357:31–7.

99. Alexander JM, Leveno KJ, Rouse DJ, et al, National Institute of Child Health and Human Development (NICHD) Maternal-Fetal Medicine Units Network (MFMU). Comparison of maternal and infant outcomes from primary cesarean delivery during the second compared with first stage of labor. Obstet Gynecol 2007;109:917–21.

100. Saunders NS, Paterson CM, Wadsworth J. Neonatal and maternal morbidity in relation to the length of the second stage of labour. Br J Obstet Gynaecol 1992;99:381–5.

101. Myles TD, Santolaya J. Maternal and neonatal outcomes in patients with a prolonged second stage of labor. Obstet Gynecol 2003;102:52–8.

102. Laughon SK, Berghella V, Reddy UM, et al. Neonatal and maternal outcomes with prolonged second stage of labor. Obstet Gynecol 2014;124:57–67.

103. Caughey AB. Is there an upper time limit for the management of the second stage of labor? Am J Obstet Gynecol 2009;201:337–8.

104. Janni W, Schiessl B, Peschers U, et al. The prognostic impact of a prolonged second stage of labor on maternal and fetal outcome. Acta Obstet Gynecol Scand 2002;81:214–21.

105. Cheng YW, Hopkins LM, Caughey AB. How long is too long: does a prolonged second stage of labor in nulliparous women affect maternal and neonatal outcomes? Am J Obstet Gynecol 2004;191:933–8.

106. Sandstrom A, Altman M, Cnattingius S, et al. Durations of second stage of labor and pushing, and adverse neonatal outcomes: a population-based cohort study. J Perinatol 2017;37:236–42.

107. Cheng YW, Hopkins LM, Laros RK Jr, et al. Duration of the second stage of labor in multiparous women: maternal and neonatal outcomes. Am J Obstet Gynecol 2007;196:585.e1-6.

108. Spong CY, Berghella V, Wenstrom KD, et al. Preventing the first cesarean delivery: summary of a joint Eunice Kennedy Shriver National Institute of Child Health and Human Development, Society for Maternal-Fetal Medicine, and American College of Obstetricians and Gynecologists Workshop. Obstet Gynecol 2012; 120:1181–93.

Labor Induction Techniques: Which Is the Best?

Christina A. Penfield, MD, MPH*, Deborah A. Wing, MD, MBA

KEYWORDS

- Labor induction • Bishop score • Prostaglandins • Foley balloon • Oxytocin
- Amniotomy

KEY POINTS

- A modified Bishop score of 6 or less is the generally accepted threshold to define an unfavorable cervix, which will benefit from cervical ripening before induction of labor.
- The most effective cervical ripening agent to achieve delivery in 24 hours is vaginal misoprostol; oral misoprostol is the most likely to achieve vaginal delivery overall.
- The combination of Foley catheter and misoprostol may be more effective than single-agent cervical ripening agents.
- The combination of amniotomy and intravenous oxytocin the most effective induction method for a favorable cervix.

INTRODUCTION

Induction of labor is the artificial stimulation of labor before its spontaneous onset to promptly achieve vaginal delivery. It is a commonly performed procedure, with approximately 1 in 5 gravid women undergoing induction of labor in both the United States and Canada in recent years.[1,2]

Induction of labor may be advisable whenever the risks of continuing the pregnancy outweigh the risks associated with induced labor and delivery. When labor induction is undertaken for appropriate reasons and with a safe and efficient approach, this procedure can greatly benefit the health of the both mothers and newborns. The indications, contraindications, and various other considerations that factor into the decision to induce labor are complex and beyond the scope of this article.

The first description of artificial induction of labor dates back to 1948 when a posterior pituitary extract of oxytocin was administered by intravenous drip for the purpose of

Disclosure Statement: Dr D.A. Wing has served as principal investigator and consultant for Ferring Pharmaceuticals, developer of the Misoprostol Vaginal Insert. She has received no financial support from this sponsor for the authorship of this report.
Department of Obstetrics and Gynecology, University of California, Irvine School of Medicine, 333 City Boulevard West, Suite 1400, Orange, CA 92868, USA
* Corresponding author.
E-mail address: christina.penfield@uci.edu

inducing labor.[3] Since then, multiple methods have been developed to recreate parturition artificially. Some methods, such as administration of ergot alkaloids, vaginal and uterine douches, and stimulant injections, have since been abandoned owing to ineffectiveness and adverse side effects, whereas other methods have withstood the test of time and continue to be used successfully in modern obstetric practice.

The modern techniques of labor induction can be divided into the following 2 broad categories depending on the status of the cervix before induction of labor.

- *Cervical ripening agents for the unfavorable cervix*: This category includes the local administration of medication, which softens and opens the cervix (prostaglandins) as well as mechanical methods, including insertion of catheters or dilators directly into the cervix.
- *Induction methods for the favorable cervix*: Administration of systemic medications that stimulate uterine contractions (ie, synthetic oxytocin) and mechanical methods such as amniotomy.

Each technique of labor induction has associated advantages and disadvantages, and as a result there is no single method that is uniformly superior for labor induction. Instead, the approach to labor induction should be tailored to the clinical scenario, with consideration given to gestational age, prior uterine surgery, fetal status, and the presence or absence of spontaneous contractions. Additionally, system factors, such as cost and the availability of immediate emergency cesarean delivery, may also weigh on the decision. Finally, an induction of labor should consider individual needs and preferences, and allow women the opportunity to make informed choices in partnership with health care providers.

ASSESSING THE CERVIX

Before starting a labor induction, the clinician must first assess the cervix to determine whether or not it is ready to start the labor process. A cervix is termed "favorable" or "ripe" to begin labor when it has softened or thinned out, making it pliable for stretching and subsequent dilation. Accurate assessment of the cervix is essential, because the selection of induction method is typically centered on the cervical status.

Bishop Score

Developed in 1964, a cervical scoring system, referred to as the Bishop score, is the most commonly used method to assess the ripeness of the cervix before induction. This system takes into account the position, consistency, effacement (shortening), and dilation of the cervix, as well as the station (location) of the presenting fetal part relative to ischial spines (**Table 1**). A modified Bishop score has also been developed that replaces effacement with cervical length.[4] In these systems, each category is assigned a score from 0 to 3, with a total maximum score of 13. A higher score reflects a cervix that is more "ripe" or "favorable" for labor induction. Traditionally, a score of 6 or less is used as a threshold to classify an "unfavorable" cervix that would benefit from cervical ripening agents during an induction of labor.[1]

In addition to determining cervical favorability, the Bishop score can also be used to predict the likelihood of vaginal delivery with induction of labor. Used in this way, a score of 6 or less is associated with a higher probability of failed induction. With a score of greater than 8, the probability of a vaginal delivery is the same for induced or spontaneous labor.[1] Aiming to make the Bishop score even more convenient, a recent study validated a simplified Bishop score using only dilation, station, and effacement. Compared with the original Bishop score cutoff of greater than 8, a

Table 1				
Modified Bishop scoring system				
	0	**1**	**2**	**3**
Dilation, cm	Closed	1–2	3–4	5–6
Effacement, %	0–30	40–50	60–70	$\geq$80
Station	−3	−2	−1, 0	+1, +2
Cervical consistency	Firm	Medium	Soft	—
Position of the cervix	Posterior	Midposition	Anterior	—

From Stock SJ, Calder AA. Induction of labour. In: Baskett TF, Calder AA, Arulkumaran S, editors. Munro Kerr's operative obstetrics. 12th edition. Edinburgh (Scottland): Elsevier; 2014. p. 71–9; with permission.

simplified Bishop score of greater than 5 has similar or better predictive ability of successful induction in a modern obstetric cohort.[5]

Transvaginal Ultrasound Imaging

Transvaginal ultrasound imaging is also used to assess cervical favorability and predict the likelihood of vaginal delivery with induction of labor. Ultrasonographic identification of a short cervical length and the presence of cervical "wedging" (any triangle "V pattern" at the area of the internal os) are considered signs of a favorable cervix. The ability of ultrasound examination to detect these early changes in the cervix, which occur before dilation, is advocated as an advantage over digital cervical assessment.[6] Additionally, transvaginal ultrasound imaging is reportedly associated with higher patient satisfaction.[7]

Using ultrasonographic signs to identify a favorable cervix may also enable providers to be more selective in their use of cervical ripening agents without adversely effecting induction outcome. Instead of using traditional Bishop score cutoffs, when a cervical length measurement of greater than 28 to 30 mm and less than 30% wedging are used as criteria for cervical ripening, the use of prostaglandins is significantly reduced without influencing vaginal delivery rates.[8,9] Ultrasound assessment, therefore, holds promise to reduce the use of cervical ripening during induction of labor, although more data are needed to confirm these results before transvaginal ultrasound imaging can be routinely recommended over the standard digital vaginal assessment.[10]

Ultrasonographic cervical length is also proposed as a method to predict mode of delivery with labor induction in term gestations, although the results are inconsistent and conflicting. The use of this modality for this purpose is, therefore, not recommended at this time.

Fetal Fibronectin

An elevated fetal fibronectin (fFN) concentration is another proposed tool to predict the duration and success of labor induction. Fibronectin is an extracellular matrix protein located in amniotic fluid and fetal membranes at the choriodecidual interface. When this interface becomes disrupted or inflamed (ie, during transformation of the cervix and membranes preceding labor) fFN "leaks" through the cervix into the vagina. Detection of this protein in cervicovaginal secretions is, therefore, associated with proximity to the onset of labor.[11–13] More recently, an elevated fFN concentration in cervicovaginal secretions at term has been associated with a shorter duration of cervical ripening and decreased time to delivery during labor induction,[11,14,15] but notably, fFN does not seem to be predictive of vaginal delivery.[15,16] Given the high cost of the fFN assay, its clinical usefulness for selecting suitable candidates for induction is limited at this time.

Summary: Cervical Assessment

- A modified Bishop score of 6 or less is the generally accepted threshold to define an unfavorable cervix, which could benefit from cervical ripening before induction of labor. A transvaginal cervical length of greater than 28 mm may also predict the need for cervical ripening.
- A simplified Bishop score of greater than 5 based on dilation, effacement, and station is predictive of vaginal delivery with induction of labor.
- The high cost and poor predictive value of fFN limit its use for predicting successful induction.

CERVICAL RIPENING WITH PHARMACOLOGIC METHODS

If the cervix is considered "unfavorable," a ripening process is generally used before labor induction. In the early 1970s, the introduction of cervical ripening methods, particularly synthetic prostaglandins, revolutionized the success of the induction process. Although considered less effective, oxytocin can also be used as a cervical ripening agent in certain clinical scenarios. Each of these options for pharmaceutical cervical ripening have distinct advantages and disadvantages in labor induction.

Prostaglandins

The administration of synthetic prostaglandins leads to changes in the cervix that mimic the natural cervical ripening process, including dissolution of collagen fibrils and increased water content that cause the cervix to swell.[17] As a result, the cervix becomes softened and distensible, and therefore more amenable to the process of thinning and dilation.[18] There are 2 synthetic prostaglandins used routinely for induction of labor: prostaglandin E1 and prostaglandin E2.

Prostaglandin E1

Misoprostol (Cytotec) is a prostaglandin E1 analog approved by the US Food and Drug Administration for the treatment and prevention of gastric ulcers related to chronic nonsteroidal antiinflammatory drug use. Administration of this drug for cervical ripening and labor induction is considered an off-label use in the United States. However, both the American College of Obstetricians and Gynecologists and Society of Obstetricians and Gynecologists of Canada consider misoprostol to be both safe and efficacious when used as a cervical ripening agent.[1,2]

Administration of prostaglandin E1 Misoprostol can be administered by vaginal, oral, and buccal/sublingual routes.

- *Vaginal administration*—The optimal dose and timing intervals of intravaginally applied misoprostol are unknown.[19–23] A metaanalysis reported that the 50-μg dose was more effective than 25 μg (eg, higher rates of delivery after a single dose, delivery within 24 hours, and a lower rate of oxytocin use), but the 25-μg dose was safer (lower rates of tachysystole, cesarean deliveries for fetal concern, neonatal intensive care unit admissions, and meconium).[24]

Recommended dosing: Lower doses, such as 25 μg, should be used initially, with redosing intervals of 3 to 6 hours.[19,25,26] The World Health Organization suggests 25 μg every 6 hours.[27]

- *Oral administration*—Oral administration of misoprostol is another option that has been evaluated in several trials. The concentration of orally administered misoprostol peaks sooner and decreases more rapidly than with vaginal administration, leading to regimens with more frequent dosing intervals.

Recommended dosing: A conservative regimen would be 50 μg tablets orally no more frequently than every 4 hours, with a maximum of 6 consecutive doses. The World Health Organization and 2 systematic reviews suggest 25 μg tablet fragments every 2 hours.[27–29]

- *Buccal or sublingual administration*—Other novel approaches to use of misoprostol, including buccal and sublingual administration, espoused for a more rapid uptake than oral or vaginal administration, have been described and have similar efficacy to vaginal routes of administration.[30–33] However, they are associated with a higher side effect profile. Therefore, more data are needed before these routes of delivery can be recommended for clinical use.

Comparisons of misoprostol use by route of delivery
- *Efficacy:* In several randomized trials, all 3 routes of administration have similar efficacy for achieving vaginal delivery within 24 hours.[30,32,34]
- *Safety:* A large systematic review found no difference in serious maternal and neonatal morbidity or death between oral and vaginal misoprostol.[28] Rates of tachysystole are similar with all 3 routes of administration. However, oral misoprostol may have a safety advantage over other routes owing to a higher consistency in dosing.
- *Patient satisfaction:* Two studies suggest that the ability to defer a digital cervical examination is considered an advantage of sublingual and oral administration,[35,36] but patient satisfaction with the various routes of administration has not been evaluated in any systematic manner.

Future prospects for misoprostol A retrievable misoprostol vaginal insert (Misodel) that delivers 200 μg over 24 hours has been developed and is available in some countries. The insert would overcome the challenges of inconsistent misoprostol dosing and allow for rapid removal with uterine tachysystole or abnormal fetal heart rate patterns. Additionally, in a large randomized trial it decreased time to onset of active labor and time to vaginal delivery compared with the dinoprostone vaginal insert.[37] Cesarean delivery rates were similar with both treatments.

Prostaglandin E2
Two prostaglandin E2 preparations containing dinoprostone are commercially available in the United States and Canada, Prepdil and Cervidil.

Prepidil This prostaglandin gel contains 0.5 mg of dinoprostone in a 2.5-mL syringe for endocervical application. If cervical change is inadequate and uterine activity is minimal after the first dose, it can be repeated every 6 to 12 hours, with no more than 1.5 mg of dinoprostone administered within a 24-hour period. Oxytocin administration should be delayed 6 to 12 hours after the final dose to avoid overstimulating the uterus.

Cervidil Cervidil is a controlled-release hydrogel pessary containing 10 mg of dinoprostone in a timed release formulation (released at a rate of 0.3 mg/h). The insert can be left in place for up to 12 hours, but should be removed if active labor begins. Oxytocin infusion can begin starting at 30 minutes after removal of the insert.

Comparison of efficacy of preparations of prostaglandin E2 A systematic review concluded that both the vaginal insert and cervical gel formulations of prostaglandin E2 have similar effectiveness in achieving active labor and vaginal delivery.[38] If regular uterine contractions are noted before the start of the induction or there is concern about the fetal heart rate pattern, use of the vaginal insert would be favored over the gel formulation because it can be discontinued if uterine tachysystole or abnormal fetal heart rate patterns develop.

Side effects of prostaglandins
Side effects of prostaglandins include tachysystole, fever, chills, vomiting, and diarrhea.

Contraindications of prostaglandins

- *Prior uterine surgery:* Prostaglandins should not be used in term pregnancies with a prior hysterotomy (ie, prior cesarean birth or myomectomy) because of the increased risk for uterine rupture.[39]
- *Preexisting uterine activity:* Baseline uterine activity is a relative contraindication to the use of prostaglandins because the addition of an exogenous uterotonic agent could lead to excessive uterine activity.
  - Consider delaying or avoiding administration in a woman with frequent, low amplitude, painless contractions or 2 or more painful contractions per 10 minutes, particularly if a uterotonic has already been administered.
  - If uterine tachysystole occurs while using prostaglandins:
    - With prostaglandin E2 (dinoprostone) vaginal insert: Remove the insert immediately.
    - With prostaglandin E1 (misoprostol) or prostaglandin E2 (dinoprostone) vaginal gel: The medication will be absorbed completely and its effect cannot be altered.
- *Concern for fetal status:* Clinicians should refrain from use of nonretrievable prostaglandins E1 and E2 vaginal gel in pregnancies with fetal heart rate abnormalities, because increased uterine activity can further compromise fetal status.

Oxytocin

Oxytocin is the most commonly used drug used to induce labor worldwide. Synthetic oxytocin is analogous to the natural oxytocin that is released from the posterior pituitary during labor, and can also promote favorable changes in the cervix. In a review of 61 studies of more than 12,000 women, oxytocin was found to be a safe method for inducing labor.[40] However, the clinical usefulness of oxytocin as a cervical ripening agent is limited by a prolonged induction time and low efficacy in achieving vaginal delivery. When comparing oxytocin with vaginal prostaglandins for third trimester cervical ripening, oxytocin leads to a lower rate of vaginal delivery within 24 hours.[40] Importantly, prolonged oxytocin use is associated with an increased risk of peripartum complications, most notably postpartum hemorrhage.[41]

Despite these disadvantages, oxytocin is the only induction agent that can be used in parturients with prior uterine surgery who desire trial of labor when mechanical methods are not feasible (ie, closed cervix). In this scenario, oxytocin can be used for cervical ripening until the cervix is dilated enough for mechanical methods.

CERVICAL RIPENING WITH MECHANICAL METHODS

Mechanical methods of induction were developed centuries ago and several of these techniques are still used commonly in modern obstetrics. These methods initiate labor by stretching the cervix, and continue to be favored owing to their low cost and lower incidence of side effects compared with other induction agents. However, the disadvantages of these techniques include discomfort with the procedure, bleeding, and risk of accidental rupture of membranes.

Membrane Stripping

In this approach, the health care provider sweeps a gloved finger over the membranes that connect the amniotic sac to the wall of the uterus. The action causes the release prostaglandins, which soften the cervix and may initiate the process of labor.[42] A systematic review found that sweeping the membranes reduced duration of pregnancy and frequency of pregnancy beyond 41 weeks.[43] This technique is therefore primarily used as a preventative strategy to avoid a formal induction of labor rather than as an induction technique itself.

Balloon Catheter

A Cook double balloon catheter specifically designed for cervical ripening is commercially available in the United States. Single balloon Foley catheters (typically #16 or #18) are also commonly used for cervical ripening. Randomized trials demonstrate similar efficacy of both single and double-balloon catheters, although the Foley catheter's low cost is a distinct advantage.

Procedure
Balloon catheters are placed using aseptic technique with continuous fetal monitoring. After placing a sterile speculum, ring forceps can be used to pass the deflated balloon catheter tip through the internal cervical os and into the extraamniotic space. If there is difficulty in passing the catheter through a narrow opening, a urologic sound can be placed inside of the catheter to direct placement. The single Foley balloon catheter is typically inflated with 30 to 60 mL of sterile water. Caution should be exercised when inflating the balloon to a high volume, because there have been sporadic reports of balloon rupture. An extraamniotic saline infusion of 30 to 40 mL/h can also be run through the catheter into the space between the internal os and placental membranes (**Fig. 1**). Data are mixed on the optimal balloon inflation volume[44,45] and appropriate duration of Foley ripening (12 vs 24 hours).[45] It is generally recommended to remove the catheter after 24 hours if it has not been spontaneously expelled.

Risk of infection
Although the balloon catheter was originally suspected to pose an increased risk of infection owing to the prolonged presence of a foreign body in the cervix, a recent large metaanalysis involving 5563 women demonstrated no increased risk of infectious morbidity associated with this technique.[46]

Future prospects for the Foley balloon catheter
Several investigators have pointed to the potential advantages of using outpatient Foley balloon ripening in uncomplicated term inductions, where the parturient returns to the hospital after a prespecified time period or when the Foley balloon is expelled. In 1 small randomized trial, the outpatient group avoided 9.6 hours of hospitalization and had similar neonatal outcomes as the group that had the Foley catheter placed while inpatient.[47] Further studies on safety and patient satisfaction are needed before this procedure can become widely implemented.

COMPARISON OF METHODS FOR CERVICAL RIPENING

When planning a labor induction, there are a multitude of available options. Taking into account considerations such as clinical history, baseline uterine activity, cervical

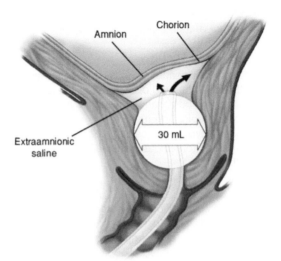

Fig. 1. Intracervical Foley balloon with extraamniotic saline infusion. (*From* Corton MM. Labor induction. In: Cunningham FG, Leveno KJ, Bloom SL, et al, editors. Williams Obstetrics, 23rd edition. New York: McGraw Hill Education; 2010; p. 504 with permission.)

examination, and fetal status should guide clinicians toward selection of the optimal cervical ripening agent (**Fig. 2**). Additionally, there is extensive research comparing the effectiveness and side effect profile of cervical ripening agents (**Table 2**).

Single-agent Methods for Cervical Ripening

When comparing methods for cervical ripening, 3 parameters are commonly used:

- Effectiveness—achieving vaginal delivery in 24 hours;
- Mode of delivery—vaginal or cesarean delivery; and
- Adverse side effects—uterine tachysystole with abnormal changes in the fetal heart rate pattern.

In a 2016 review of 96 randomized trials, the authors compared single-agent methods for cervical ripening and concluded that no method of cervical ripening demonstrates superiority in every parameter.[48] Instead, a different agent excelled in each of the 3 categories. Vaginal misoprostol was the most effective agent, with the highest likelihood of achieving vaginal delivery in 24 hours. Meanwhile, oral misoprostol was associated with the highest likelihood of vaginal delivery overall. These 2 findings were confirmed in another recent systematic review and network metaanalysis of 611 studies.[49]

In these systematic reviews, vaginal and sublingual/buccal misoprostol had the highest incidence of uterine hyperstimulation.[49] In contrast, the induction agent with the least adverse side effects was the Foley catheter.[48] Therefore, the preferred induction agent should be selected based on relative preference for effecting delivery within 24 hours, minimizing tachysystole and other fetal side effects, and avoiding a cesarean delivery.

Combination Methods for Cervical Ripening

Given that mechanical and pharmacologic cervical ripening agents have different mechanisms of action, it is plausible that using these methods simultaneously could produce synergistic effects. Combination methods typically use Foley catheter with simultaneous administration of either prostaglandins or oxytocin infusions.

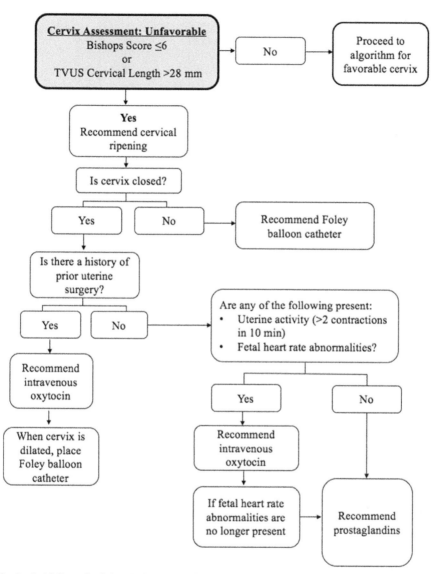

Fig. 2. Guidelines for labor induction with an unripe cervix. TVUS, transvaginal ultrasound imaging.

The most promising combination method for cervical ripening is Foley catheter and misoprostol. Although preliminary studies did not detect an advantage to using Foley catheter and prostaglandins together over using these agents individually, these trials were limited by small sample size, different dosing of misoprostol, and heterogeneous labor management.[50–52] More recently, 2 large randomized studies demonstrated that the combination of Foley and either oral or vaginal misoprostol reduced time to delivery compared with vaginal misoprostol alone.[53,54] In another recent randomized study, women who received both Foley catheter and vaginal misoprostol were twice as likely to deliver earlier than women who received Foley or vaginal misoprostol alone.[55]

Table 2
Comparison of cervical ripening agents

Agent	Advantages	Disadvantages	Best Practice	Cost[a]
Oxytocin	• Ability to titrate dosage quickly with abnormal fetal heart rate pattern • Ability to precisely titrate its effect	• Increased time from induction to vaginal delivery compared with other agents	• Cervical ripening in trial of labor after cesarean when cervix is closed.	10-mL ampule $53.31
Prostaglandin E1 (misoprostol)	• Decreased time to delivery • Highest rates of vaginal delivery overall	• Contraindicated in the setting of prior uterine surgery • Higher rates of uterine tachystole • Avoid use in the setting of preexisting uterine activity or concern for potential fetal decompensation owing to inability to reverse uterine stimulation	• Cervical ripening with closed cervix • Adjunct to mechanical methods	100-µg tab = $1.09
Prostaglandin E2 vaginal insert (Cervidil)	• Ability to reverse uterine stimulation after administration • May be used in cases where fetus is stable but there is concern for potential decompensation	• Increased time from administration to delivery • Discouraged in the setting of preexisting uterine activity or abnormal fetal status	• Cervical ripening in a closed cervix when fetus is stable but there is concern for potential decompensation	$218.94
Mechanical methods (Foley balloon, Cooks Foley balloon)	• Ability to reverse uterine stimulation after administration • May be used in cases where fetus is stable but there is concern for potential decompensation	• Discomfort with procedure	• Cervical ripening in cervix that is minimally dilated • May consider adding vaginal misoprostol simultaneously	Foley balloon $3.00 Cook Foley balloon $41.00

[a] This cost in US dollars is an estimate of the wholesale cost and does not include the cost of the entire induction or the hospital markup.

The other option for dual cervical ripening, Foley catheter and oxytocin infusion, has not demonstrated consistent benefit over Foley catheter alone. In two older randomized trials, the addition of oxytocin to Foley catheter did not significantly reduce likelihood of delivery within 24 hours, total time to delivery, or vaginal delivery rate.[55,56] In contrast, three more recent large randomized trials demonstrated reduced time to delivery with Foley catheter induction when oxytocin infusion was infused simultaneously.[55,57,58] Due to these conflicting reports, more studies are needed to confirm efficacy before this combination cervical ripening method can be recommended universally.

Only one randomized study compared the two dual cervical ripening regimens head-to-head; this study demonstrated that the misoprostol and Foley combination significantly reduced time to delivery compared to combining Foley catheter and oxytocin together.[55]

Summary: Comparison of Cervical Ripening Methods

- Most effective agent: Vaginal misoprostol.
- Most likely to achieve vaginal delivery: Oral misoprostol.
- Least adverse side effects: Foley catheter.
- The combination of Foley catheter and misoprostol appears to be more effective than single-agent cervical ripening in several randomized controlled trials.

INDUCTION TECHNIQUES FOR THE FAVORABLE CERVIX

If the cervix is favorable, cervical ripening agents are not typically necessary, and instead the use of intravenous oxytocin and artificial rupture of membranes is preferred. Several clinical considerations, such as parity and fetal station, should factor into the decision for which method should be used first—oxytocin, amniotomy, or a combination of the both methods simultaneously (**Fig. 3**).

Mechanical Methods for Induction in the Favorable Cervix: Amniotomy

Artificial rupture of membranes is a procedure used to intentionally rupture the chorioamniotic membranes with the goal to induce or augment labor. To rupture membranes, the cervix must be dilated, typically to at least 3 cm. To minimize the risk of umbilical cord prolapse after rupture of membranes, the fetal vertex should not be floating and must be well-applied to the cervix. The amniotomy procedure is typically carried out by an Amnihook, which is used to create a small opening in the membranes. The fetal heart rate should be monitored before and after membrane rupture.

Timing of amniotomy
There is concern that earlier rupture of membranes will lead to an overall longer exposure to ruptured membranes during labor, which has the potential to increase risk of chorioamnionitis. Therefore, the appropriate timing of artificial rupture of the membranes that balances the risk of infection with the benefits of expedited labor induction is debated. In a randomized trial of nulliparous women undergoing induction of labor, women randomized to rupture of membranes at 4 cm (vs >4 cm) had shortened time to delivery without an increase in maternal or neonatal infectious complications.[59] However, early amniotomy did not decrease the risk of cesarean delivery.

Addition of oxytocin to amniotomy
When amniotomy is used to induce labor, the combination of amniotomy with intravenous oxytocin is more effective than amniotomy alone.[60] For women with a favorable cervix, this combination is more successful than other agents in achieving vaginal delivery in 24 hours.[49]

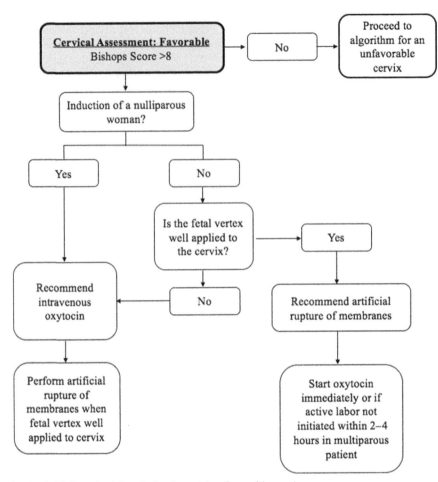

Fig. 3. Guidelines for labor induction with a favorable cervix.

However, there may be clinical scenarios, such as an induction of labor for a multiparous woman with a favorable cervix, where amniotomy alone may also be effective.[61] We recommend either starting oxytocin immediately with artificial rupture of membranes, or if active labor does not start within 2 to 4 hours after amniotomy in a multiparous patient.

Summary: amniotomy

- Artificial rupture of membranes should only be performed when the fetal vertex is well-applied to the cervix. Performing amniotomy at 4 cm may shorten time to delivery without increasing the risk of infection.
- The combination of amniotomy and intravenous oxytocin is the most effective induction method for a favorable cervix.

Pharmacologic Methods in the Favorable Cervix: Oxytocin

Oxytocin induces biochemical changes in uterine myofibrils and increases local prostaglandin production to further stimulate uterine contractions. Its synthetic analog Pitocin or Syntocinon is typically administered by intravenous infusion for labor induction with a favorable cervix. A commonly used strategy is to begin the induction with oxytocin until artificial rupture of membranes is feasible and the vertex is well-applied to the cervix.

Table 3 Oxytocin protocols			
	Starting Dose (mU/min)	Incremental Dose Increase (mU/min)	Dosage Interval (min)
Low dose	0.5–1	1	30–40
Alternative low dose	1–2	2[a]	15–30
High dose	6	6	15–40
Alternative high dose	4	4	15

[a] The incremental increase should be reduced to 3 mU/min if tachysystole is present, and reduced to 1 mU/min if recurrent hyperstimulation. Some clinicians limit to a maximum cumulative dose of 10 U and a maximum duration of 6 hours.

Oxytocin protocols

The goal of oxytocin infusion is to stimulate sufficient uterine activity to dilate the cervix and produce fetal descent without causing hypertonic contractions of the uterus, which can decrease oxygenation of the fetus and, rarely, result in uterine rupture. To achieve this delicate balance, several protocols for oxytocin administration have been developed (**Table 3**). The aim of these protocols is to increase oxytocin dosing until strong contractions occurring every 2 to 3 minutes are achieved, or uterine activity the reaches 200 to 250 Montevideo units, as measured by an intrauterine pressure catheter. These regimens seem to be similar in achieving vaginal delivery in 24 hours.[62] Although the high-dose regimen may decrease time to delivery, it is also associated with higher rates of tachysystole (albeit without an increase in maternal and perinatal complications).[62]

The plasma half-life of oxytocin is short, with a uterine response in 3 to 6 minutes, and a steady concentration of oxytocin in plasma is achieved by 40 minutes with continuous infusion.[63] This allows for relatively quick titration to achieve adequate uterine stimulation and also enables the clinician to abruptly discontinue uterine stimulation if tachysystole an abnormal fetal heart rate pattern develop.

SUMMARY

This article presented an evidence-based overview of contemporary methods available for labor induction. Familiarity with the advantages and disadvantages of these methods for various clinical scenarios will guide clinicians toward an induction plan that is safe, effective, and patient centered, and achieve the overall goal of a healthy mother and newborn.

REFERENCES

1. ACOG Committee on Practice Bulletins – Obstetrics. ACOG Practice Bulletin No. 107: induction of labor. Obstet Gynecol 2009;114(2 Pt 1):386–97.
2. Leduc D, Biringer A, Lee L, et al, Society of Obstetricians and Gynaecologists of Canada. Induction of labour. J Obstet Gynaecol Can 2013;35(9):840–60.
3. Theobald GW, Graham A. The use of post-pituitary extract in physiological amounts in obstetrics; a preliminary report. Br Med J 1948;2(4567):123–7.
4. Brennand JE, Calder AA. Labor and normal delivery: induction of labor. Curr Opin Obstet Gynecol 1991;3(6):764–8.
5. Laughon SK, Zhang J, Troendle J, et al. Using a simplified Bishop score to predict vaginal delivery. Obstet Gynecol 2011;117(4):805–11.
6. Boozarjomehri F, Timor-Tritsch I, Chao CR, et al. Transvaginal ultrasonographic evaluation of the cervix before labor: presence of cervical wedging is associated with shorter duration of induced labor. Am J Obstet Gynecol 1994;171(4):1081–7.

7. Tan PC, Vallikkannu N, Suguna S, et al. Transvaginal sonographic measurement of cervical length vs. Bishop score in labor induction at term: tolerability and prediction of Cesarean delivery. Ultrasound Obstet Gynecol 2007;29(5):568–73.

8. Bartha JL, Romero-Carmona R, Martínez-Del-Fresno P, et al. Bishop score and transvaginal ultrasound for preinduction cervical assessment: a randomized clinical trial. Ultrasound Obstet Gynecol 2005;25(2):155–9.

9. Park KH, Kim SN, Lee SY, et al. Comparison between sonographic cervical length and Bishop score in preinduction cervical assessment: a randomized trial. Ultrasound Obstet Gynecol 2011;38(2):198–204.

10. Ezebialu IU, Eke AC, Eleje GU, et al. Methods for assessing pre-induction cervical ripening. Cochrane Database Syst Rev 2015;(6):CD010762. Ezebialu IU, ed.

11. Blanch G, Oláh KS, Walkinshaw S. The presence of fetal fibronectin in the cervicovaginal secretions of women at term–its role in the assessment of women before labor induction and in the investigation of the physiologic mechanisms of labor. Am J Obstet Gynecol 1996;174(1 Pt 1):262–6.

12. Lockwood CJ, Senyei AE, Dische MR, et al. Fetal fibronectin in cervical and vaginal secretions as a predictor of preterm delivery. N Engl J Med 1991; 325(10):669–74.

13. Nageotte MP, Casal D, Senyei AE. Fetal fibronectin in patients at increased risk for premature birth. Am J Obstet Gynecol 1994;170(1 Pt 1):20–5.

14. Garite TJ, Casal D, Garcia-Alonso A, et al. Fetal fibronectin: a new tool for the prediction of successful induction of labor. Am J Obstet Gynecol 1996;175(6): 1516–21.

15. Sciscione A, Hoffman MK, DeLuca S, et al. Fetal fibronectin as a predictor of vaginal birth in nulliparas undergoing preinduction cervical ripening. Obstet Gynecol 2005;106(5 Pt 1):980–5.

16. Reis FM, Gervasi MT, Florio P, et al. Prediction of successful induction of labor at term: role of clinical history, digital examination, ultrasound assessment of the cervix, and fetal fibronectin assay. Am J Obstet Gynecol 2003;189(5):1361–7.

17. Word RA, Li X-H, Hnat M, et al. Dynamics of cervical remodeling during pregnancy and parturition: mechanisms and current concepts. Semin Reprod Med 2007;25(1):69–79.

18. Keirse MJNC. Natural prostaglandins for induction of labor and preinduction cervical ripening. Clin Obstet Gynecol 2006;49(3):609–26.

19. Hofmeyr GJ, Gülmezoglu AM, Pileggi C. Vaginal misoprostol for cervical ripening and induction of labour. Cochrane Database Syst Rev 2010;(10):CD000941.

20. Wing DA, Ortiz-Omphroy G, Paul RH. A comparison of intermittent vaginal administration of misoprostol with continuous dinoprostone for cervical ripening and labor induction. Am J Obstet Gynecol 1997;177(3):612–8.

21. Farah LA, Sanchez-Ramos L, Rosa C, et al. Randomized trial of two doses of the prostaglandin E1 analog misoprostol for labor induction. Am J Obstet Gynecol 1997;177(2):364–9 [discussion: 369–71].

22. Wing DA. Labor induction with misoprostol. Am J Obstet Gynecol 1999;181(2): 339–45.

23. Sanchez-Ramos L, Kaunitz AM. Misoprostol for cervical ripening and labor induction: a systematic review of the literature. Clin Obstet Gynecol 2000;43(3):475–88.

24. McMaster K, Sanchez-Ramos L, Kaunitz AM. Balancing the efficacy and safety of misoprostol: a meta-analysis comparing 25 versus 50 micrograms of intravaginal misoprostol for the induction of labour. BJOG 2015;122(4):468–76.

25. Calder AA, Loughney AD, Weir CJ, et al. Induction of labour in nulliparous and multiparous women: a UK, multicentre, open-label study of intravaginal misoprostol in comparison with dinoprostone. BJOG 2008;115(10):1279–88.
26. Tan T-C, Yan SY, Chua TM, et al. A randomised controlled trial of low-dose misoprostol and dinoprostone vaginal pessaries for cervical priming. BJOG 2010; 117(10):1270–7.
27. Tang J, Kapp N, Dragoman M, et al. WHO recommendations for misoprostol use for obstetric and gynecologic indications. Int J Gynaecol Obstet 2013;121(2):186–9.
28. Alfirevic Z, Aflaifel N, Weeks A. Oral misoprostol for induction of labour. Cochrane Database Syst Rev 2014;(6):CD001338.
29. Kundodyiwa TW, Alfirevic Z, Weeks AD. Low-dose oral misoprostol for induction of labor: a systematic review. Obstet Gynecol 2009;113(2 Pt 1):374–83.
30. Souza A, Amorim M, Feitosa F. Comparison of sublingual versus vaginal misoprostol for the induction of labour: a systematic review. BJOG 2008;115(11):1340–9.
31. Wolf SB, Sanchez-Ramos L, Kaunitz AM. Sublingual misoprostol for labor induction: a randomized clinical trial. Obstet Gynecol 2005;105(2):365–71.
32. Shetty A, Mackie L, Danielian P, et al. Sublingual compared with oral misoprostol in term labour induction: a randomised controlled trial. BJOG 2002;109(6): 645–50.
33. Shetty A, Danielian P, Templeton A. Sublingual misoprostol for the induction of labor at term. Am J Obstet Gynecol 2002;186(1):72–6.
34. Elhassan EM, Nasr AM, Adam I. Sublingual compared with oral and vaginal misoprostol for labor induction. Int J Gynaecol Obstet 2007;97(2):153–4.
35. Nassar AH, Awwad J, Khalil AM, et al. A randomised comparison of patient satisfaction with vaginal and sublingual misoprostol for induction of labour at term. BJOG 2007;114(10):1215–21.
36. Zahran KM, Shahin AY, Abdellah MS, et al. Sublingual versus vaginal misoprostol for induction of labor at term: a randomized prospective placebo-controlled study. J Obstet Gynaecol Res 2009;35(6):1054–60.
37. Wing DA, Brown R, Plante LA, et al. Misoprostol vaginal insert and time to vaginal delivery: a randomized controlled trial. Obstet Gynecol 2013;122(2 Pt 1):201–9.
38. Thomas J, Fairclough A, Kavanagh J, et al. Vaginal prostaglandin (PGE2 and PGF2a) for induction of labour at term. Cochrane Database Syst Rev 2014;(6):CD003101.
39. Lydon-Rochelle M, Holt VL, Easterling TR, et al. Risk of uterine rupture during labor among women with a prior cesarean delivery. N Engl J Med 2001;345(1):3–8.
40. Alfirevic Z, Kelly AJ, Dowswell T. Intravenous oxytocin alone for cervical ripening and induction of labour. Cochrane Database Syst Rev 2009;(4):CD003246.
41. Grotegut CA, Paglia MJ, Johnson LNC, et al. Oxytocin exposure during labor among women with postpartum hemorrhage secondary to uterine atony. Am J Obstet Gynecol 2011;204(1):56.e1-6.
42. McColgin SW, Bennett WA, Roach H, et al. Parturitional factors associated with membrane stripping. Am J Obstet Gynecol 1993;169(1):71–7.
43. Boulvain M, Stan C, Irion O. Membrane sweeping for induction of labour. Cochrane Database Syst Rev 2005;(1):CD000451.
44. Delaney S, Shaffer BL, Cheng YW, et al. Labor induction with a Foley balloon inflated to 30 mL compared with 60 mL: a randomized controlled trial. Obstet Gynecol 2010;115(6):1239–45.
45. Gu N, Ru T, Wang Z, et al. Foley catheter for induction of labor at term: an open-label, randomized controlled trial. PLoS One 2015;10(8):e0136856.

46. McMaster K, Sanchez-Ramos L, Kaunitz AM. Evaluation of a transcervical Foley catheter as a source of infection. Obstet Gynecol 2015;126(3):539–51.
47. Sciscione AC, Muench M, Pollock M, et al. Transcervical Foley catheter for preinduction cervical ripening in an outpatient versus inpatient setting. Obstet Gynecol 2001;98(5 Pt 1):751–6.
48. Chen W, Xue J, Peprah MK, et al. A systematic review and network meta-analysis comparing the use of Foley catheters, misoprostol, and dinoprostone for cervical ripening in the induction of labour. BJOG 2016;123(3):346–54.
49. Alfirevic Z, Keeney E, Dowswell T, et al. Methods to induce labour: a systematic review, network meta-analysis and cost-effectiveness analysis. BJOG 2016; 123(9):1462–70.
50. Chung JH, Huang WH, Rumney PJ, et al. A prospective randomized controlled trial that compared misoprostol, Foley catheter, and combination misoprostol-Foley catheter for labor induction. Am J Obstet Gynecol 2003;189(4):1031–5.
51. Rust OA, Greybush M, Atlas RO, et al. Preinduction cervical ripening. A randomized trial of intravaginal misoprostol alone vs. a combination of transcervical Foley balloon and intravaginal misoprostol. J Reprod Med 2001;46(10):899–904.
52. Barrilleaux PS, Bofill JA, Terrone DA, et al. Cervical ripening and induction of labor with misoprostol, dinoprostone gel, and a Foley catheter: a randomized trial of 3 techniques. Am J Obstet Gynecol 2002;186(6):1124–9.
53. Carbone JF, Tuuli MG, Fogertey PJ, et al. Combination of Foley bulb and vaginal misoprostol compared with vaginal misoprostol alone for cervical ripening and labor induction: a randomized controlled trial. Obstet Gynecol 2013;121(2 Pt 1):247–52.
54. Hill JB, Thigpen BD, Bofill JA, et al. A randomized clinical trial comparing vaginal misoprostol versus cervical Foley plus oral misoprostol for cervical ripening and labor induction. Am J Perinatol 2009;26(1):33–8.
55. Levine LD, Downes KL, Elovitz MA, et al. Mechanical and pharmacologic methods of labor induction: a randomized controlled trial. Obstet Gynecol 2016;128(6):1357–64.
56. Pettker CM, Pocock SB, Smok DP, et al. Transcervical Foley catheter with and without oxytocin for cervical ripening: a randomized controlled trial. Obstet Gynecol 2008;111(6):1320–6.
57. Connolly KA, Kohari KS, Rekawek P, et al. A randomized trial of Foley balloon induction of labor trial in nulliparas (FIAT-N). Am J Obstet Gynecol 2016;215(3): 392.e1–6.
58. Schoen CN, Grant G, Berghella V, et al. Intracervical Foley catheter with and without oxytocin for labor induction. Obstet Gynecol 2017;129(6):1046–53.
59. Macones GA, Cahill A, Stamilio DM, et al. The efficacy of early amniotomy in nulliparous labor induction: a randomized controlled trial. Am J Obstet Gynecol 2012;207(5):403.e1-5.
60. Howarth GR, Botha DJ. Amniotomy plus intravenous oxytocin for induction of labour. Cochrane Database Syst Rev 2001;(3):CD003250.
61. Tan PC, Soe MZ, Sulaiman S, et al. Immediate compared with delayed oxytocin after amniotomy labor induction in parous women: a randomized controlled trial. Obstet Gynecol 2013;121(2 Pt 1):253–9.
62. Budden A, Chen LJY, Henry A. High-dose versus low-dose oxytocin infusion regimens for induction of labour at term. Cochrane Database Syst Rev 2014;(10):CD009701.
63. Seitchik J, Amico J, Robinson AG, et al. Oxytocin augmentation of dysfunctional labor. IV. Oxytocin pharmacokinetics. Am J Obstet Gynecol 1984;150(3):225–8.

Is There a Place for Outpatient Preinduction Cervical Ripening?

 CrossMark

Beth Leopold, MD, Anthony Sciscione, DO*

KEYWORDS

• Outpatient • Preinduction • Cervical ripening • Safety

KEY POINTS

• Induction of labor continues to be one of the most commonly performed tasks in obstetrics.
• Strategies to improve patient/family satisfaction, decrease resource allocation along with costs, and assure safety will be paramount.
• Although there are many potential candidates, it seems that outpatient preinduction cervical ripening with the Foley catheter meets these criteria in a properly selected group of low-risk women.

INTRODUCTION

The rate of induction of labor more than doubled between 1990 and 2010 going from 9.6% to 23.7%. The rate of induction has stayed steady with the rate in 2014 being 23.2% for all races according to the National Vital Statistics.[1] Reasons for induction range from intrauterine growth restriction, gestational diabetes, preeclampsia, and postdates. There are many strategies for induction including pharmacologic and mechanical methods. Women who undergo induction frequently have an unfavorable cervix. Generally, an unfavorable cervix refers to a cervix that is close, posterior, firm, and not effaced. A Bishops score of less than 6 is usually considered an unfavorable cervix.[2] Labor induction, particularly in nulliparous women, can take an extended period and can be achieved through various pharmaceutical and mechanical methods. Replacing inpatient induction with outpatient strategies continues to be attractive for physicians, midwives, nurses, and hospital administrators. Decreasing length of hospital stays, cost, and workload and increasing satisfaction and number of vaginal deliveries is favorable and continues to be studied. This article reviews the different methods, safety, and efficacy of outpatient cervical ripening techniques.

Department of Obstetrics and Gynecology, Christiana Care Health System, 4755 Ogletown-Stanton Road, PO BOX 6001, Newark, Delaware 19718, USA
* Corresponding author.
E-mail address: asciscione@christianacare.org

Obstet Gynecol Clin N Am 44 (2017) 583–591
http://dx.doi.org/10.1016/j.ogc.2017.08.010
0889-8545/17/© 2017 Elsevier Inc. All rights reserved.

obgyn.theclinics.com

METHODS
Foley Bulb

The technique of Foley balloon for induction of labor was first described in 1860s.[3] The Foley catheter is a relatively inexpensive and effective method used to perform mechanical cervical ripening. The Foley catheter works through mechanical dilation of the cervix as it is extruded. With dilation of the cervix, endogenous prostaglandins are released that further augment cervical ripening.[4] The Foley catheter comes in multiple sizes, but the Foley catheter works by having the catheter threaded through the cervix, inflating the balloon so that it sits just past the internal os, and taping the catheter to the patient's leg on tension. Multiple studies are looking at various aspects of the Foley catheter for cervical ripening including how much to inflate the balloon, whether to put the Foley bulb on tension, and when and which pharmaceutical induction agents should be used to reduce cesarean delivery rates and time to delivery. Studies show that Foley bulbs are more effective than placebo in cervical ripening.[5,6] Sciscione and colleagues[7] in 2001 found that in 111 women randomly assigned to either 30-mL Foley catheter or 50 μg every 4 hours of vaginal misoprostol, Foley catheters are equally as likely to result in vaginal delivery as vaginal misoprostol and that time to delivery is not significantly different. A recent meta-analysis by Fox and colleagues[8] found that the Foley catheter resulted in fewer contractile abnormalities and less meconium passage.

Outpatient data

Sciscione and colleagues,[9] in a prospective trial, looked at outpatient versus inpatient Foley balloon induction of labor. These authors randomly selected 61 full-term women with vertex presentations, reactive nonstress test, appropriate amniotic fluid index, with a Bishop score less than 5. They found that Foley bulb was as effective in the outpatient setting as in the inpatient setting for preinduction cervical ripening. Furthermore, they found that maximum dose of oxytocin, time of oxytocin, epidural rate, induction time, Apgar scores, and cord pH levels were not significantly different. Importantly, the outpatient group had 9.6 fewer hours of hospital time. A pilot randomized, controlled trial from Wilkinson and colleagues[10] looked at 48 women randomly assigned to either outpatient or inpatient Foley catheter insertion. Although the study was not powered to measure significant differences in rates of cesarean delivery, infection, or delivery within 24 hours, they did find a significant reduction in the total amount of oxytocin used for the outpatient Foley catheter group. They found a 24% reduction in total oxytocin used in the outpatient group. They proposed that the ability to go home and physically relax allowed women to be more likely to go into labor naturally after Foley catheter placement. It is clear that the Foley catheter can be effectively managed by a patient in the outpatient setting.

Risks and safety profile

Overall, Foley balloons are a safe form of cervical ripening. Sciscione and colleagues[11] gauged safety by retrospectively reviewing women in the inpatient setting and applied an outpatient Foley balloon protocol. They found that adverse events including cesarean delivery for nonreassuring fetal heart tracing, abruption and intrapartum still birth were not increased in the study group. There were no cesarean deliveries for those reasons in the 1905 patients who met inclusion criteria. The 3 cesarean deliveries that occurred during the study periods were 1 for face presentation and 2 for arrest of dilation. These 3 women also went into labor naturally or had rupture of membranes during the study period, which would have excluded them from the outpatient protocol.[11]

There is a theoretic risk that Foley balloon placement will increase the risk of intrapartum intrauterine infection. A 2015 meta-analysis from McMaster and colleagues[12] looked at 26 randomized, controlled trials that included 5563 women undergoing induction of labor through either prostaglandin preparations or Foley catheter placement. They found that there was no significant difference in rates of chorioamnionitis between the 2 groups. In 2004, a study looked at rates of intrauterine infection comparing inpatient and outpatient Foley balloon placement. This study found that there was no difference in infection rates between the inpatient and outpatient groups.[13] With the American College of Obstetrics and Gynecology's replacing chorioamnionitis with intra-amniotic infection and inflammation (Triple I), new studies are needed to reassess the rates of infection between prostaglandin formulations and Foley catheter insertion.

Prostaglandin Gel and Insert

Background

Similar to the Foley catheters, vaginal prostaglandins and inserts have been used since the 1960s.[14,15] Prostaglandins work by directly ripening the cervix through enzymatic degradation of collagen and increasing the water content of the extracellular matrix. They also indirectly stimulate the myometrium to induce contractions.[2] There are 2 formulations of prostaglandin E2 (PGE2) that are currently available: dinoprostone gel that comes in a 2.5-mL syringe with 0.5 mL of dinoprostone and a vaginal insert containing 10 mg of dinoprostone. Kho and colleagues[16] and D'Aniello and colleagues[17] compared the 2 formulations for effectiveness and safety profiles. They both found that neither formulation preformed better in reducing time to delivery, rates of cesarean delivery, or any other birth outcome. Contrarily, Ashwal and colleagues[18] found that a vaginal PGE2 insert achieved more cervical ripening and shorter subsequent time to delivery than the vaginal gel. Overall, dinoprostone was found to be more effective than placebo or no treatment in reducing time to vaginal delivery. In particular, Thomas and colleagues[19] found that PGE2 probably increases the chance of vaginal delivery within 24 hours, but that it also increases the chances of uterine hyperstimulation and subsequent fetal heart rate changes from 1% to 5%.

Outpatient data

Much of the initial data about outpatient cervical ripening came from PGE2 gels and inserts. PGE2 has been found to be effective in the outpatient setting. O'Brien and colleagues[20] found in a randomized, double-blind, placebo-controlled trial that 2 mg PGE2 vaginal gel daily for up to 5 consecutive days was more efficacious than placebo in reducing time to delivery and had higher rates of admissions for spontaneous labor. Patients were observed for the first 30 minutes after vaginal gel placement. They found that only one patient out of 100 low-risk patients had tachysystole, which did not require intervention. Similarly, McKenna and colleagues[21] studied at women at 38 weeks or greater with a Bishop score of less than 9 who received either intracervical prostaglandin gel or placebo for induction in the outpatient setting. They found that 50% delivered within 2 days in the study group compared with only 16% in the placebo group.

When compared with PGE2 in the inpatient setting, outpatient PGE2 was found have no effect on time to delivery but to have higher rates of satisfaction than the inpatient group. In Biem and colleagues,[22] 300 full-term women were randomly assigned to either inpatient or outpatient PGE2 for induction of labor. They found that the women in the outpatient group had a 56% rate of high satisfaction compared with only 39% in the inpatient group, despite having similar pain and anxiety levels.

The OPRA study, also by Wilkinson and colleagues[23] looked at 827 women randomly assigned to inpatient versus outpatient vaginal PGE2 induction of labor. They measured rates of delivery within 24 hours, oxytocin use, rate of cesarean delivery, and epidural use and found no significant differences between any of these measures.

Other studies looked at the cost effectiveness of outpatient PGE2 induction protocols. Farmer and colleagues[24] found in 1996 that the outpatient group accrued significant less costs than the inpatient ($3835.00 ± 2172.00 vs $5049.00 ± 2060.00) and significant less time in the hospital (74.4 ± 33.1 hours vs 100.3 ± 41.6 hours). Importantly, they showed that no differences in maternal or fetal outcomes including cesarean delivery rates or neonatal intensive care unit (NICU) admission would have changed costs significantly. A more recent cost analysis in 2013 from Adelson and colleagues[25] found that in an Australian trial comparing inpatient and outpatient PGE2 protocols, there were no significant cost savings in the outpatient group.

Risk and safety profile
The risk of hyperstimulation and subsequent nonreassuring fetal heart rate with vaginal PGE2 is one of the reasons many obstetricians worry about outpatient PGE2 without continuous or intermittent monitoring. The National Institute for Health and Care Excellence (NICE) guidelines still allow for vaginal PGE2 use in the outpatient setting with continued auditing of the induction. However, other groups have come out against vaginal PGE2 in the outpatient setting for cervical ripening, as they are worried about contractions that can be caused by PGE2 and the possibility of nonreassuring fetal heart rate tracing (NRFHT) without monitoring in the outpatient setting.

Salvador and colleagues[26] performed a large retrospective cohort trial that looked at more than 1300 women who underwent either inpatient or outpatient induction with dinoprostone. They found no differences in fetal outcomes, including 5-minute Apgar scores or NICU admissions.[26] In the Kelly and colleagues[14] study, there were no significant differences between maternal or fetal outcomes. Contrarily, the OPRA study, discussed above, found that there was an increased rate of tachysystole and NRFHT in the group randomly assigned to outpatient induction in the initial hour-long monitoring period. More than half of the patients randomly assigned to this group were either not allowed to actually be discharged to home secondary to fetal heart rate concerns or patient anxiety or the patient returned to the hospital before the prearranged time because of concerns about labor. Similarly, Tassone and colleagues[27] looked at 111 women who underwent cervical ripening with sustained vaginal PGE2 insert and were monitored in the hospital for 12 hours in a simulated outpatient setting. They found that 23.4% ended up having regular contractions and that 27.9% removed the vaginal insert before the end of the 12 hours. The authors concluded that the use of this vaginal insert may not be favorable in the outpatient setting given the high rate of uterine contractions and removal of the insert.

Cytotec

Background
Cytotec, or misoprostol, is a synthetic PGE1 that can be given bucally, sublingually, vaginally, or rectally for cervical ripening. It was originally marketed in 1988 for gastric ulcers as a cytoprotective agent. Since the early 1990s, studies have found that it is effective in cervical ripening and labor induction in full-term pregnancies.[2] American Congress of Obstetricians and Gynecologists Practice Bulletin 107 on induction of labor states that despite the off-label use of misoprostol, it is recommended for cervical ripening.[28] A 2010 Cochrane review showed that vaginal misoprostol was more effective than Foley catheters, vaginal PGE2 inserts or gels, oxytocin, or placebo alone for

cervical ripening. This analysis found a higher rate of uterine tachysystole and cesarean deliveries for NRFHTs but fewer for failure of labor progression.[29]

Multiple studies compared misoprostol with one specific other induction mechanism. Fox and colleagues[8] looked at 9 prospective, randomized, controlled trials including 1603 patients comparing Foley catheter and intravaginal misoprostol for cervical ripening. Their meta-analysis found no significant differences in mean time to delivery, rate of cesarean deliveries, and chorioamnionitis. When comparing misoprostol and PGE2, Austin and colleagues[30] found that women who received misoprostol had higher rates of vaginal delivery within 12 and 24 hours compared with dinoprostone.

Outpatient data

Oral and vaginal misoprostol have been studied for cervical ripening in the outpatient setting. Compared with placebo, 25 µg of vaginal misoprostol was found to be more effective in causing women to enter into a regular contraction pattern within 48 hours. Stitely and colleagues[31] looked at women who received 25 µg of vaginal misoprostol in the morning for 2 days, and if they did not go into labor by the third day, they were scheduled for inpatient induction. They found the reduction in necessity of induction on day 3 from 84.8% to 11.1%. In 2004, another study by McKenna and colleagues[32] looked at 25 µg of vaginal misoprostol and randomly assigned 68 women to either study group or placebo group. They found that a single dose of 25 µg of vaginal misoprostol was effective in reducing time to delivery in full-term gestations with unfavorable cervices. Similarly, PonMalar and colleagues[33] in 2017 looked at 126 women randomly assigned to either 25 µg of vaginal misoprostol compared with placebo and also found that misoprostol decreased time to delivery.

Gaffaney and colleagues[34,35] changed the route of delivery of the misoprostol but still looked at misoprostol compared with placebo. They found that 100 µg of oral misoprostol daily for 3 days decreased time to delivery compared with placebo without subsequent increases in poor maternal or neonatal outcomes.

Chang and colleagues[36] compared 50 µg of vaginal misoprostol and administration in the outpatient and inpatient setting. They gave the patient 1 dose of 50 µg of misoprostol either in the inpatient setting or outpatient setting and were instructed to return to the hospital the next morning for continuation of their labor induction. The outpatient group was found to be further dilated at the time of admission the next morning and had decreased time from admission to delivery. This study was not powered to observe adverse outcomes.

Meyer and colleagues[37] found that when comparing cytotec in the outpatient setting with dinoprostone, misoprostol reduced the overall dose of oxytocin, time of oxytocin administration, and maximum dose of oxytocin.

Risk and safety

There is a significant risk of uterine tachysystole with misoprostol administration. Fox and colleagues[8] found a significantly higher rate of uterine tachysystole in the women treated with misoprostol. Similarly, in the PROBAAT-M trial, misoprostol had higher rates of tachysystole with and without NRFHT than Foley catheter. However, there were no significant differences in Apgar scores or NICU admissions.[38] Similarly Austin and colleagues[30] found higher rates of uterine tachysystole without concomitant decrease in Apgar scores or increased rates of NICU admission. In most studies, hospital staff monitors patients before discharge to continue their inductions in the outpatient setting. Patients are not allowed to go home if they experience uterine tachysystole, NRFHT, or painful contractions.

Nitric Oxide

Background

Nitric oxide donors have also been used for cervical ripening. This method works by softening the cervix by rearranging cervical collagen and ground collagen.[2] Research has looked mostly at outpatient administration of isosorbide mononitrate administration in the outpatient setting before admission for continuation of labor induction. Studies in the inpatient setting have mostly compared nitric oxide donors to other forms of induction. The PRIM study from 2006 compared vaginal isosorbide mononitrate with PGE2 vaginal gel. This study found that although cervical ripening worked better with prostaglandins, patients were more satisfied with isosorbide mononitrate.[39] Collingham and colleagues[40] compared vaginal misoprostol with vaginal misoprostol plus isosorbide mononitrate. They found that there was no additional benefit of vaginal isosorbide mononitrate to vaginal misoprostol for decreasing time to delivery. Overall, nitric oxide donors are an attractive option for the outpatient setting given that their risk of tachysystole and subsequent NRFHT is significantly less.

Outpatient data

Multiple studies looked at vaginal isosorbide mononitrate for labor induction in the outpatient setting. Habib and colleagues[35] performed at randomized, double-blind, placebo-controlled trial in which they gave 102 women either vaginal isosorbide mononitrate or placebo and measured time to delivery from administration. They found that the study group had a shorter time to delivery with fewer study patients needing prostaglandins for labor induction. Bullarbo and colleagues,[41] similarly, randomly assigned 200 women at 42 weeks gestation to either 40 mg isosorbide mononitrate or placebo in the outpatient setting. They found that of the women who did not go into labor naturally, the time to deliver of the study group and placebo group were not statistically different. The IMOP study looked at self-administered vaginal isosorbide mononitrate compared with placebo in the outpatient setting. They found that isosorbide mononitrate did not shorten time to delivery compared with placebo.[42] Similarly the NOCETER study did not show decreased times to delivery.[43]

Risk and safety profile

Nitric oxide donors primarily work by ripening the cervix and not by inducing labor. A 2011 Cochrane review reported on the safety of nitric oxide donors in the outpatient setting. They reviewed 19 studies that compared isosorbide mononitrate with either placebo or another method of induction. The review found that although isosorbide mononitrate is relatively safe compared with other methods of induction in the outpatient setting, it is less effective. There were fewer patients of uterine hyperstimulation without NRFHTs but increased numbers of patients still pregnant between 24 and 48 hours and more patients with an unfavorable cervix between 12 and 24 hours compared with those with vaginal misoprostol.[14] More studies are needed to further evaluate the use of isosorbide mononitrate's safety in combination with other cervical ripening techniques in the outpatient setting.

SUMMARY

Induction of labor continues to be one of the most commonly performed tasks in obstetrics. If trials like the National Institute of Child Health and Human Development's ARRIVE trial find that delivery for all women at 39 weeks provides a significant advantage in pregnancy outcomes, the number of women who will require induction of labor will significantly increase. Regardless, strategies to improve patient/family satisfaction, decrease resource allocation along with costs, and assure safety will be paramount. Although there are many potential candidates, it appears that outpatient preinduction cervical ripening with the Foley catheter meets these criteria in a properly selected group of low-risk women.

REFERENCES

1. Hamilton BE, Martin JA, Osterman MJ, et al. National vital statistics reports. Natl Vital Stat Rep 2015;64(12):1–64.
2. Amorosa JM, Stone JL. Outpatient cervical ripening. Semin Perinatol 2015;39: 488–94. Elsevier; 2015.
3. Smith JA. Balloon Dilators for Labor Induction: a Historical Review. J Med Ethics Hist Med 2013;6:10.
4. Thiery M. Ripening procedures: European Association of Gynaecologists and Obstetricians: 2nd Meeting, Paris, 4–5 September, 1987. Eur J Obstet Gynecol Reprod Biol 1988;28(2):95–102.
5. Jozwiak M, Bloemenkamp KW, Kelly AJ, et al. Mechanical methods for induction of labour. Cochrane Database Syst Rev 2012;(3):CD001233.
6. Vaknin Z, Kurzweil Y, Sherman D. Foley catheter balloon vs locally applied prostaglandins for cervical ripening and labor induction: a systematic review and metaanalysis. Am J Obstet Gynecol 2010;203(5):418–29.
7. Sciscione AC, Nguyen L, Manley J, et al. A Randomized Comparison of Transcervical Foley Catheter to Intravaginal Misoprostol for Preinduction Cervical Ripening. Obstet Gynecol 2001;97(4):603–7.
8. Fox N, Saltzman D, Roman A, et al. Intravaginal misoprostol versus Foley catheter for labour induction: a meta-analysis. BJOG 2011;118(6):647–54.
9. Sciscione AC, Muench M, Pollock M, et al. Transcervical Foley catheter for preinduction cervical ripening in an outpatient versus inpatient setting. Obstet Gynecol 2001;98(5):751–6.
10. Wilkinson C, Adelson P, Turnbull D. A comparison of inpatient with outpatient balloon catheter cervical ripening: a pilot randomized controlled trial. BMC Pregnancy Childbirth 2015;15(1):126.
11. Sciscione AC, Bedder CL, Hoffman MK, et al. The timing of adverse events with Foley catheter preinduction cervical ripening; implications for outpatient use. Am J Perinatol 2014;31(09):781–6.
12. McMaster K, Sanchez-Ramos L, Kaunitz AM. Evaluation of a Transcervical Foley Catheter as a Source of Infection: A Systematic Review and Meta-analysis. Obstet Gynecol 2015;126(3):539–51.
13. McKenna DS, Duke JM. Effectiveness and infectious morbidity of outpatient cervical ripening with a Foley catheter. J Reprod Med 2004;49(1):28–32.
14. Kelly AJ, Malik S, Smith L, et al. Vaginal prostaglandin (PGE2 and PGF2a) for induction of labour at term. Cochrane Database Syst Rev 2009;(4):CD003101.
15. Kelly AJ, Munson C, Minden L. Nitric oxide donors for cervical ripening and induction of labour. Cochrane Database Syst Rev 2011;(6):CD006901.
16. Kho EM, Sadler L, McCOWAN L. Induction of labour: A comparison between controlled-release dinoprostone vaginal pessary (Cervidil®) and dinoprostone intravaginal gel (Prostin E2®). Aust N Z J Obstet Gynaecol 2008;48(5):473–7.
17. D'Aniello G, Bocchi C, Florio P, et al. Cervical ripening and induction of labor by prostaglandin E2: a comparison between intracervical gel and vaginal pessary. J Matern Fetal Neonatal Med 2003;14(3):158–62.

18. Ashwal E, Hiersch L, Melamed N, et al. Pre-induction cervical ripening: comparing between two vaginal preparations of dinoprostone in women with an unfavorable cervix. J Matern Fetal Neonatal Med 2014;27(18):1874–9.
19. Thomas J, Fairclough A, Kavanagh J, et al. Vaginal prostaglandin (PGE2 and PGF2a) for induction of labour at term. Cochrane Database Syst Rev 2014;(6):CD003101.
20. O'brien JM, Mercer BM, Cleary NT, et al. Efficacy of outpatient induction with low-dose intravaginal prostaglandin E2: a randomized, double-blind, placebo-controlled trial. Am J Obstet Gynecol 1995;173(6):1855–9.
21. McKenna DS, Costa SW, Samuels P. Prostaglandin E2 cervical ripening without subsequent induction of labor. Obstet Gynecol 1999;94(1):11–4, 19.
22. Biem SR, Turnell RW, Olatunbosun O, et al. A randomized controlled trial of outpatient versus inpatient labour induction with vaginal controlled-release prostaglandin-E 2: effectiveness and satisfaction. J Obstet Gynaecol Can 2003;25(1): 23–31.
23. Wilkinson C, Bryce R, Adelson P, et al. A randomised controlled trial of outpatient compared with inpatient cervical ripening with prostaglandin E2 (OPRA study). BJOG 2015;122(1):94–104.
24. Farmer KC, Schwartz WJ, Rayburn WF, et al. A cost-minimization analysis of intracervical prostaglandin E2 for cervical ripening in an outpatient versus inpatient setting. Clin Ther 1996;18(4):747–56.
25. Adelson PL, Wedlock GR, Wilkinson CS, et al. A cost analysis of inpatient compared with outpatient prostaglandin E 2 cervical priming for induction of labour: results from the OPRA trial. Aust Health Rev 2013;37(4):467–73.
26. Salvador SC, Simpson ML, Cundiff GW. Dinoprostone vaginal insert for labour induction: a comparison of outpatient and inpatient settings. Journal of Obstetrics and Gynaecology Canada 2009;31(11):1028–34.
27. Tassone SA, Pearman CR, Rayburn WF. Outpatient cervical ripening using a sustained-release prostaglandin E2 vaginal insert. The Journal of reproductive medicine 2001;46(6):599.
28. ACOG Practice Bulletin No. 107: Induction of Labor. Obstet Gynecol 2009; 114(2, Part 1):386–97.
29. Hofmeyr GJ, Gülmezoglu AM. Vaginal misoprostol for cervical ripening and induction of labour. Cochrane Database Syst Rev 2003;(1):CD000941.
30. Austin SC, Sanchez-Ramos L, Adair CD. Labor induction with intravaginal misoprostol compared with the dinoprostone vaginal insert: a systematic review and metaanalysis. Am J Obstet Gynecol 2010;202(6):624.e1-9.
31. Stitely ML, Browning J, Fowler M, et al. Outpatient cervical ripening with intravaginal misoprostol. Obstet Gynecol 2000;96(5):684–8, 27.
32. McKenna DS, Ester JB, Proffitt M, et al. Misoprostol outpatient cervical ripening without subsequent induction of labor: a randomized trial. Obstet Gynecol 2004;104(3):579–84.
33. PonMalar J, Benjamin SJ, Abraham A, et al. Randomized double-blind placebo controlled study of preinduction cervical priming with 25 μg of misoprostol in the outpatient setting to prevent formal induction of labour. Arch Gynecol Obstet 2017;295(1):33–8.
34. Gaffaney CAL, Saul LL, Rumney PJ, et al. Outpatient oral misoprostol for prolonged pregnancies: a pilot investigation. Am J Perinatol 2009;26(09):673–7.
35. Habib SM, Emam SS, Saber AS. Outpatient cervical ripening with nitric oxide donor isosorbide mononitrate prior to induction of labor. Int J Gynecol Obstetrics 2008;101(1):57–61.

36. Chang DW, Velazquez MD, Colyer M, et al. Vaginal Misoprostol for Cervical Ripening at Term: Comparison of Outpatient vs. Inpatient Administration. Obstet Gynecol Surv 2006;61(3):167–8.
37. Meyer M, Pflum J, Howard D. Outpatient misoprostol compared with dinoprostone gel for preinduction cervical ripening: a randomized controlled trial. Obstet Gynecol 2005;105(3):466–72.
38. Jozwiak M, ten Eikelder M, Rengerink KO, et al. Foley catheter versus vaginal misoprostol: randomized controlled trial (PROBAAT-M study) and systematic review and meta-analysis of literature. Am J Perinatol 2014;31(02):145–56.
39. Osman I, MacKenzie F, Norrie J, et al. The "PRIM" study: a randomized comparison of prostaglandin E 2 gel with the nitric oxide donor isosorbide mononitrate for cervical ripening before the induction of labor at term. Am J Obstet Gynecol 2006;194(4):1012.
40. Collingham JP, Fuh KC, Caughey AB, et al. Oral misoprostol and vaginal isosorbide mononitrate for labor induction: a randomized controlled trial. Obstet Gynecol 2010;116(1):121–6.
41. Bullarbo M, Orrskog ME, Andersch B, et al. Outpatient vaginal administration of the nitric oxide donor isosorbide mononitrate for cervical ripening and labor induction postterm: a randomized controlled study. Am J Obstet Gynecol 2007; 196(1):50.e1-5.
42. Bollapragada S, MacKenzie F, Norrie J, et al. Randomised placebo-controlled trial of outpatient (at home) cervical ripening with isosorbide mononitrate (IMN) prior to induction of labour–clinical trial with analyses of efficacy and acceptability. The IMOP Study. BJOG 2009;116(9):1185–95.
43. Schmitz T, Fuchs F, Closset E, et al. Outpatient cervical ripening by nitric oxide donors for prolonged pregnancy: a randomized controlled trial. Obstet Gynecol 2014;124(6):1089–97.

Augmentation of Labor

A Review of Oxytocin Augmentation and Active Management of Labor

Annessa Kernberg, MD*, Aaron B. Caughey, MD, PhD

KEYWORDS

• Augmentation • Oxytocin • Oxytocin protocol • Cesarean

KEY POINTS

• Augmentation of labor may reduce cesarean delivery.
• Active management of labor may reduce cesarean delivery.
• Active management of labor shortens the length of labor.
• Specific oxytocin protocols are increasingly used to standardize care.

INTRODUCTION

Augmentation of labor is the process of increasing the frequency and/or strength of contractions to facilitate a faster labor or to more readily achieve a vaginal delivery. Although augmentation may be achieved through natural means, in particular nipple stimulation, as well as artificial rupture of the membranes, the principal method that varies in its use and approach is via oxytocin infusion. Oxytocin is widely used for both induction and augmentation of labor. Historically, in the 1950s, oxytocin utilization increased as du Vigneaud and colleagues[1] synthesized an exogenous version, enabling increased administrative control and, therefore, decreasing potential risks. Oxytocin has known risks, including uterine tachysystole (more than 5 contractions per 10 minutes), which has been associated with a lower umbilical artery pH at birth and may affect maternal cardiovascular and renal systems.[2–4] Even with these known risks, a strict predictable administrative protocol does not exist and medication use has risen as induction of labor rates have increased. Induction of labor rates nearly tripled, with estimates rising from 9.6% to 23.2% of deliveries from 1990 to 2014.[5] Although induction of labor is a common procedure, the process varies considerably. Initiation doses range from 0.5 mU/min to 6 mU/min and increments from 1 mU/min to

Disclosure Statement: The authors do not have any commercial or financial conflicts of interest.
Department of Obstetrics and Gynecology, Oregon Health & Science University, 3181 Southwest Sam Jackson Park Road, Portland, OR 97239-3098, USA
* Corresponding author. Department of Obstetrics and Gynecology, Oregon Health & Science University, 3181 Southwest Sam Jackson Park Road, Mail code – L466, Portland, OR 97239-3098.
E-mail address: Kernberg@OHSU.edu

Obstet Gynecol Clin N Am 44 (2017) 593–600
http://dx.doi.org/10.1016/j.ogc.2017.08.012
0889-8545/17/© 2017 Elsevier Inc. All rights reserved.

obgyn.theclinics.com

6 mU/min, with maximum dosing from 16 mU/min to 117 mU/min nd and increment intervals from 15 minutes to 60 minutes.[6] Similarly, oxytocin augmentation protocols vary in their dosing regimens.

BACKGROUND

In the 1960s, O'Driscoll and colleagues[7] pioneered the active management of labor (AML). The optimal goal was a vaginal delivery within 12 hours of admission. Carefully outlining the protocol, the investigators included labor diagnosis, early amniotomy, high-dose oxytocin, and continuous labor support. The oxytocin dosage included an initial dose of 10 drops and increased every 15 minutes to a maximum of 60 drops per minute. These values in today's language translate to an initial dose of 4 mU/min and incremental increase every 15 minutes to a maximum of 40 mU/min. In 1973, this approach proved successful in a prospective trial of 1000 women, with only 7 women undelivered after 12 hours. Based on this information, O'Driscoll and colleagues[7] confidently wrote, "it is possible to regulate the duration [of labor] with almost complete success. This requires a systematic approach with formal diagnosis, regular assessment, and decisive action in every case"—a powerful statement fueling more than 50 years of continued research in optimizing active management, minimizing potential harm, and decreasing operative deliveries. Nearly a decade later in 1987 another prospective randomized study by Cohen and colleagues[8] evaluated whether aggressive management of labor lowered cesarean deliveries. The results were less optimistic because management did not change the mode of delivery or perinatal outcomes, and on top of that the duration of labor was not significantly shortened. Torn between dichotomous results, active management was criticized. The next step involved protocol dissemblance, assessing each augmentation component (amniotomy and oxytocin) critically, and reevaluating outcomes (duration of labor vs cesarean section rates).

In the 1990s several important large clinical trials of AML were published. The 2 largest showed a significant reduction in labor lasting greater 12 hours, from 19% to 5%[9] and from 26% to 9%.[10] The oxytocin protocol studied by López-Zeno and colleagues[9] involved an initial dose of 6 mU/min and increased every 15 minutes, with a maximum of 36 mU/min. In a slightly less aggressive approach, but consistent with O'Driscoll's oxytocin protocol, Frigoletto and colleagues[10] used an oxytocin protocol involving an initial dose of 4 mU/min and increased by 4 mU/min every 15 minutes, with a maximum of 40 mU/min. Both the studies differed regarding the effects of cesarean section rates, with López-Zeno and colleagues[9] demonstrating a 26% reduction and Frigoletto and colleagues[10] demonstrating no difference. Even with these 2 large, randomized trials, questions about the potential impact of AML continued. Do the differing oxytocin regimens make a difference or does amniotomy with early cervical dilation have a greater impact? — certainly 9 have been suggested and studied (**Table 1**)? In terms of neonatal outcomes, it is reassuring that meta-analyses have not found an association between oxytocin use and neonatal outcomes regarding Apgar scores, neonatal ICU admission, neurologic abnormalities, or umbilical cord gases.[11] In 2013, a Cochrane review of high-dose and lose-dose oxytocin regimens echoed these outcomes, finding no significant differences in Apgar scores or umbilical cord pH, although high-dose regimens reduced rate of cesarean sections (relative risk [RR] 0.62; 95% CI, 0.44–0.86) and increased vaginal birth (RR 1.35; 95% CI, 1.13–1.62).[12]

Without question, further research is needed to determine the optimal benefit of oxytocin while also minimizing potential risk. Although AML protocols looked at rapid increases of oxytocin, there was less of a focus on minimizing risks. Approaches that take a more balanced perspective often use checklists or have several items designed

Table 1
Active management of labor — oxytocin protocols

Source	Initial Dose (mU/min)	Interval Time (min)	Increment (mU/min)	Maximum (mU/min)
ACOG[15]	Low: 0.5–2 High: 6	15–40	Low: 1–2 High: 3–6	Not reported
O'Driscoll et al,[7] 1973	4	15	Not reported	40
Frigoletto et al,[10] 1995	4	15	4	40
López-Zeno et al,[9] 1992	6	15	Not reported	36
Bor et al,[16]	3.3	20	3.3	30
Rossen et al,[17] 2016	6	15	3	40
Nippita et al,[20] 2017	1–2.5	Not reported	Not reported	16, 32, 40
Hehir et al,[21] 2017	5	15	5	30
Kenyon et al,[12] 2013	Low: 1–2 High: 4–7	15–40	Low: <4 High: ≥4	Not reported

to also decrease or stop the oxytocin infusion. In 2007, Clark and colleagues[13] conducted a retrospective review and data extraction examining the effects of a checklist-based protocol for oxytocin administration centered on maternal and fetal response to medical administration rather than infusion rate. Examination of 100 patients before and after the use of an oxytocin checklists revealed 17% reduction in maximum infusion rates (13.8 mU/min vs 11.4 mU/min) without lengthening time to delivery (8.5 hours vs 8.2 hours) and overall cesarean delivery rate declined (15% vs 13%). The preoxytocin checklist consisted of 12 points, which ensured assessment and documentation of maternal and fetal status, physical examination findings, and the ability to perform a cesarean section if indicated. During oxytocin administration, an in-use checklist consisted of fetal assessment based on fetal heart monitoring and uterine assessment based on tocometer and palpation between contractions. The study involved 125 obstetric facilities in 20 states allowing for generalizability. Uniform oxytocin mixing and infusion were implemented throughout the study sites but were not outlined in the article. Clark and colleagues[13] emphasized the need to improve patient safety while maximizing success of delivery. The subsequent cascade of research in this area similarly emphasized patient safety, as seen in 2008 with the Hayes and Weinstein[14] literature review on optimizing oxytocin administration while minimizing side effects. The suggested protocol consisted of an initial dose of 2 mU/min (12 mL/h) and incremental increase of 2 mU every 45 minutes until adequate labor, with a maximum dose of 16 mU/min.[14] Within the American College of Obstetricians and Gynecologists (ACOG) practice bulletin number 107,[15] last updated August 2009, each hospital's individual department should develop guidelines regarding oxytocin administration. Examples of low-dose and high-dose oxytocin protocols are then outlined. The low-dose protocol involves an initial dose of 0.5 mU/min to 2 mU/min and incremental increase of 1 mU/min to 2 mU/min every 15 minutes to 40 minutes. The high-dose protocol involves an initial dose of 6 mU/min and incremental increase of 3 mU/min to 6 mU/min every 15 minutes to 40 minutes. Maximal doses are not established.[15] These protocols were based on data extracted from studies dating back to 1986 and even among these recommendations a wide range of initial dose, incremental increase, and intervals between titration exist. To improve patient safety, greater uniformity of care and standardization of protocols, including initial dose, incremental increase, and interval time between doses, are warranted.

LITERATURE REVIEW

To identify recent research on oxytocin protocols, the authors conducted a literature review of studies over the past 1.5 years (2016–2017). The keywords, oxytocin, Pitocin, labor, induction of labor, protocol, and augmentation, were used in PubMed. The analysis initially identified 1431 articles but selected a subset of 6 specifically pertaining to an oxytocin augmentation protocol. Of these articles, 2 were retrospective cohort studies, 2 reviews, 1 a randomized controlled trial, and 1 a prospective trial. The following section reviews these articles temporally.

As discussed previously, and found in this literature review, oxytocin protocols vary considerable with an initial dose of 1 mU/min to 7 mU/min, incremental increase of 1 mU/min to 6 mU/min every 15 minutes to 40 minutes, and maximum doses from 16 mU/min to 40 mU/min (see **Table 1**). The following is a review of the 6 studies in chronically order starting with the oldest.

Few studies have reviewed the duration of oxytocin use and the potential for minimizing the duration of use to minimize associated risks. Discontinuing oxytocin administration is a potential method to shorten exposure length but may subsequently affect labor length. Bor and colleagues[16] in a randomized controlled trial investigated whether discontinuation of oxytocin infusion increased the length of the active phase of labor; 200 women with an initial cervical dilatation of less than or equal to 4 cm were randomized to either continue or discontinue oxytocin infusion when cervical dilation reached 5 cm. The primary outcome was the time from 5 cm to delivery. Results illustrated a prolonged active phase by 41 minutes (95% CI) in the discontinued group versus the continuous group (median 125 minutes vs 88 minutes) in women who reached active phase and delivered vaginally. Higher, although not statistically significant, was the incidence of tachysystole, cesarean deliveries, postpartum hemorrhage, third-degree perineal laceration, and adverse neonatal outcomes. The oxytocin protocol consisted of an initial dose of 3.3 mU/min and incremental increase of 3.3 mU/min every 20 minutes, with a maximum dose of 30 mU/min.[16] The study was a randomized controlled trial, which is a strength. Limitations include noncompliance among the discontinuation group, and 64% of women were restarted on oxytocin even when there was progression of labor based on cervical dilation. Therefore, results are difficult to interpret.

Rossen and colleagues,[17] in a prospective trial, implemented an oxytocin protocol, which outlined criteria for initiation and subsequently assessed maternal and neonatal outcomes. From January 2009 to December 2013, data from 20,227 deliveries were collected. The women either presented in spontaneous labor or underwent induction without a previous cesarean section. Prior to 2010, oxytocin was administered if the provider thought that labor was progressing slowly. The protocol was implemented in 2010 and defined prolonged labor as lack of cervical dilation after 4 hours from previous assessment, which is consistent with World Health Organization partograph.[18] Subsequent oxytocin administration consisted of an initial dose of 6 mU/min and incremental increase of 3 mU/min every 15 minutes, with a maximum dose of 40 mU/min; 3926 deliveries encompassed the preprotocol group, with the remainder 16,301 in the postprotocol group. Results showed a decrease in augmentation with an associated decrease in frequency of emergency cesarean section from 6.9% to 5.3%. In nulliparous women undergoing induction of labor, the emergent cesarean section rate declined from 26.5% to 15.7%; fourth-degree lacerations also decreased from 5.6% to 1.2%. Umbilical cord was collected and the frequency of infants with pH less than 7.1 reduced from 4.7% to 3.2% but did not reach statistical significance with a pH less than 7.0.[17] Strengths in this study include the large population size, the use of a standardized oxytocin protocol, education, clear definition of prolonged labor, and the implementation of monthly quality assurance throughout the study. The study was observational, and duration of oxytocin use or maximum doses were not captured along with rates of chorioamnionitis, therefor, contributing to the study's limitations. The study highlights the importance of oxytocin protocols to ensure clear definitions, accurate assessment, and clinical reasoning with implementation.

Duration between dose adjustments was the focus of Loscul and colleagues'[19] retrospective review of 454 primiparous women in spontaneous labor. The group was subdivided into oxytocin adjustment with increments less than 20 minutes versus greater than 20 minutes, with postpartum hemorrhage as the primary outcome. Obstetric and neonatal outcomes were analyzed; 43.8% of the women's oxytocin was increased in less than 20 minutes, and in turn these women had higher rates of postpartum hemorrhage (6.5% vs 3.5%). This relationship remained significant after adjusting for risk factors. Apgar score less than or equal to 7 at 5 minute of life or pH less than or equal to 7.10 was worse in the less than 20-minute interval group (12.1% vs 4.3%). The investigators, therefore, concluded a minimal oxytocin interval should be 20 minutes. Strengths of the study include the ability to obtain this level of detail regarding oxytocin administration as well as the ability to assess umbilical artery pH. The study only assessed primiparous women in spontaneous labor, which limits generalizability.

In New South Wales, Australia, in 2011, an oxytocin protocol was mandated. Nippita and colleagues[20] surveyed 66 New South Wales hospitals to assess changes in clinical practice preprotocol (2008) and post-protocol (2014). In 2008 within-district hospitals, there were 11 minimum initial oxytocin doses (range: 0.25–6.67 mU/min) and 13 maximums (4–40 mU/mL). In 2014, there were only 2 initial oxytocin doses (1.0 mU/min or 2.5 mU/min) and 3 maximums (1640 mU/min, 3240 mU/min, or 40 mU/min). The results illustrate a shift toward standardized protocols. The ability to obtain information from a large group of hospitals is strength of the study. Limitations do exist because only 64% of hospital participated in 2014, and, therefore, information regarding the remainder was not obtained, leading to selection bias. The survey was self-reported, and, therefore, actual adherence to the protocol was not examined. Lastly, maternal and neonatal outcomes before and after the implementation of the protocol were not examined. In the end, the study is an evaluation of policy change.

In a retrospective cohort study, Hehir and colleagues[21] examined the outcomes of vaginal birth after cesarean section (VBAC) presenting in spontaneous labor with implementation of a standardized intrapartum protocol. The protocol outlined AML, which included but was not limited to the following: early amniotomy, 1-to-1 midwifery care, continuous fetal monitoring, 2-hour interval assessment, and team communication. The obstetrician is informed when a patient with a history of cesarean section is laboring. Expected rate of change was 1 cm/h. Otherwise, oxytocin augmentation was indicated with consultation from the obstetrician. Oxytocin administration consisted of an initial dose of 5 mU/min and incremental increase of 5 mU/min every 15 minutes, with a maximum dose of 30 mU/min; 2222 secundiparous women from 2001 to 2011 underwent a trial of labor after a cesarean (TOLAC) and presented in spontaneous labor; 72.5% (1611/2222) of these women had a successful VBAC and 27.5% (611/2222) underwent a repeat intrapartum cesarean section. Maternal and neonatal outcomes were then compared between these groups. With regard to maternal outcomes, the following were present in only the intrapartum cesarean group: 12 cases of uterine rupture (incidence of 0.54%). Both groups had 2 peripartum hysterectomies (incidence of 0.18%). There was 1 maternal death in the setting of an unknown placenta accreta after VBAC. Infants delivered via cesarean section were more likely to have an Apgar score of less than 7 at 5 minutes (1.5% vs 0.5%; odds ratio [OR] 3.0; 95% CI, 1.2–7.8) but were not more likely to have an arterial pH less than 7.0 (2.0% vs 1.0%; OR 2.1; 95% CI, 0.67–6.8). One infant born with a pH of 6.7 died in the first 24 hours of life although mode of delivery was not reported.[21] Hehir and colleagues[21] demonstrate that VBAC is obtainable with a standardized protocol in place. Strengths of the study include the large cohort of women, standardization of oxytocin administration over a 10-year period, and the ability to evaluate maternal and neonatal mortality. Limitations in the study include the inability to assess indications for cesarean section and to assess outcomes before and after implementation of the intrapartum protocol and, therefore, it is unclear if the differences in outcomes reflect protocol utilization or differences in 2 groups.

Lastly, Kenyon and colleagues[12] conducted a review of randomized and quasirandomized controlled trials comparing initial dose and incremental increase of oxytocin in women undergoing labor augmentation with high-dose or low-dose regimens. High-dose regimens were defined as an initial dose or incremental increase of 4 mU/min or more. Low-dose regimens were defined as an initial dose or incremental increase of less than 4 mU/min. Incremental intervals were 15 minutes to 40 minutes for both regimens. Four studies of 664 women demonstrated high-dose regimens reduced duration of labor (mean difference −3.50 hours; 95% CI, −6.38 to −0.62), reduced rate of cesarean section (RR 0.62; 95% CI, 0.44–0.86), and increased vaginal birth (RR 1.35; 95% CI, 1.13–1.62). No significant differences were found between the regimens for operative vaginal deliveries, epidural placement, postpartum hemorrhage, chorioamnionitis, Apgar scores, or umbilical cord pH. Perinatal mortality, uterine rupture, and other outcomes were not evaluated. The investigators, therefore, concluded there is insufficient evidence to recommend high-dose regimens. Among the included studies, the investigators analyzed risk of bias, including allocation, blinding, incomplete outcome data, and selective reporting, which is a strength of the study. The review process is affected by selection bias from the investigators, because Kenyon, as an author of the article, was also an investigator of 1 of the included trials, which is a limitation of the study. Also the article did not outline the maximum oxytocin dose and if that value differs between the 2 regimens. Overall, the results demonstrate a difference of outcomes between regimens and further studies are needed.

SUMMARY

There is a wide range of approaches to the management of augmentation of labor with oxytocin. There are ranges in both the dosing of oxytocin and in how it is chosen for use and identified to decrease or stop the dosing. It seems that oxytocin use is a part of a program that reduces cesarean delivery; however, on its own, the best evidence only supports that its use reduces the length of labor. The focus on safety over the past decade and going forward is dependent on standardized use of oxytocin through the use of checklists, protocols, or both. Such approaches have included discontinuation of oxytocin once cervical change is assessed, criteria for oxytocin initiation, and intervals between dose adjustments. Over time, as investigators report implementation of protocols, intrapartum protocols may improve maternal and neonatal outcomes for those undergoing augmentation in a variety of settings, and high-dose regimens may reduce duration of labor and cesarean deliveries. Randomized controlled trials and prospective, natural experiments and cohort studies are needed in the effort to create the evidence base to understand how standardized protocols may be used to ensure greater patient safety while improving all obstetric outcomes.

REFERENCES

1. du Vigneaud V, Ressler C, Swan J, et al. The synthesis of an octapeptide amide with the hormonal activityof oxytocin. J Am Chem Soc 1953;75(19):4879–80.
2. Svanstrom MC, Biber B, Hanes M, et al. Signs of myocardial ischemia after injection of oxytocin: a randomized double-blind comparision of oxytocin and methylergometrine during cesarean section. Br J Anaesth 2008;100(5):683–9.
3. Bakker PC, Kurver PH, Kuik DJ, et al. Elevated uterine activity increased the risk of fetal acidosis at birth. Am J Obstet Gynecol 2007;196(4):313.e1-6.
4. Li C, Wang W, Summer S, et al. Molecular mechanisms of antidiuretic effect of oxytocin. J Am Soc Nephrol 2008;19(2):225–32.
5. Hamilton BE, Martin JA, Osterman MJK, et al. Births: final data for 2014. Natl Vital Stat Rep 2015;64(12):1–64.
6. Cunningham FG. Induction of labour. In: Cunningham FG, Leveno KJ, Bloom SL, et al, editors. Williams obstetrics. New York: McGraw Hill; 2010. p. 540–1.
7. O'Driscoll K, Stronge JM, Minogue M. Active management of labour. Br Med J 1973;3(5872):135–7. Available at: http://www.ncbi.nlm.nih.gov/pmc/articles/PMC1586344/.
8. Cohen GR, O'Brien WF, Lewis L, et al. A prospective randomized study of the aggressive management of early labor. Am J Obstet Gynecol 1987;157(5):1174–7.
9. López-Zeno JA, Peaceman AM, Adashek JA, et al. A controlled trial of a program for the active management of labor. N Engl J Med 1992;326(7):450–4.
10. Frigoletto FD Jr, Lieberman E, Lang JM, et al. A clinical trial of active management of labor. N Engl J Med 1995;333(12):745–50.
11. Fraser W, Vendittelli F, Krauss I, et al. Effects of early augmentation of labour with amniotomy and oxytocin in nulliparous women: a meta-analysis. Br J Obstet Gynaecol 1998;105(2):189–94.
12. Kenyon S, Tokumasu H, Dowswell T, et al. High-dose versus low-dose oxytocin for augmentation of delayed labour. Cochrane Database Syst Rev 2013;(7). CD007201. Available at: http://onlinelibrary.wiley.com/doi/10.1002/14651858.CD007201.pub3/abstract.
13. Clark S, Belfort M, Saade G, et al. Implementation of a conservative checklist-based protocol for oxytocin administration: maternal and newborn outcomes. Am J Obstet Gynecol 2007;197(5):480.e1-5.
14. Hayes EJ, Weinstein L. Improving patient safety and uniformity of care by a standardized regimen for the use of oxytocin. Am J Obstet Gynecol 2008;198(6):622.e1-7.
15. American College of Obstetricians and Gynecologists. ACOG practice bulletin no. 107: induction of labor. Obstet Gynecol 2009;114(2 pt 1):286–397.
16. Bor P, Ledertoug S, Boie S, et al. Continuation versus discontinuation of oxytocin infusion during the active phase of labour: a randomised controlled trial. BJOG: An International Journal of Obstetrics & Gynaecology 2016;123(1):129–35.
17. Rossen J, Østborg TB, Lindtjørn E, et al. Judicious use of oxytocin augmentation for the management of prolonged labor. Acta Obstet Gynecol Scand 2016;95(3):355–61.
18. WHO recommendations for augmentation of labour. 2014. Available at: http://www.who.int/reproductivehealth/publications/maternal_perinatal_health/augmentationlabour/en/. Retrieved July 25, 2017.

19. Loscul C, Chantry A-A, Caubit L, et al. Association between oxytocin augmentation intervals and the risk of postpartum haemorrhage. J Gynecol Obstet Biol Reprod (Paris) 2016;45(7):708–15 [in French].

20. Nippita TAC, Roberts CL, Nicholl MC, et al. Induction of labour practices in New South Wales Hospitals: before and after a statewide policy. Aust N Z J Obstet Gynaecol 2017;57(1):111–4.

21. Hehir MP, Mackie A, Robson MS. Simplified and standardized intrapartum management can yield high rates of successful VBAC in spontaneous labor. J Matern Fetal Neonatal Med 2017;30(12):1504–8.

Elective Induction of Labor

What is the Impact?

Sarah E. Little, MD, MPH

KEYWORDS

- Elective induction • Non–medically indicated induction • Induction of labor
- Cesarean delivery

KEY POINTS

- Elective induction (induction without maternal/fetal indication) is not associated with an increased risk of cesarean delivery compared with expectant management of pregnancy.
- Elective induction after 39 weeks may be associated with decreased maternal morbidity (such as infection) and decreased neonatal morbidity (such as respiratory distress).
- Recent reductions in elective early term delivery do not seem to have significantly increased stillbirth rates; however, elective induction after 39 weeks may theoretically lower the risk of stillbirth.
- Elective induction may be associated with increased resource use and cost, decreased patient satisfaction, and lower rates of breastfeeding.

INTRODUCTION

Labor induction is a common intervention in the United States, occurring in nearly a quarter of births.[1] There are a broad range of medical indications for induction, which are typically recommended to prevent worsening maternal disease, neonatal morbidity, or fetal death. Elective inductions are those without any medical indication in healthy women with a singleton pregnancy. Some researchers and policy experts advocate calling these non–medically indicated inductions, rather than elective inductions; however, these two terms are used fairly interchangeably.[2–4] Elective delivery before 39 weeks is associated with increased neonatal morbidity[5] and elective inductions are not recommended before 39 weeks.[3] Thus, this article reviews the impact of inductions after 39 weeks, and more specifically at 39 or 40 weeks' gestation, because many providers recommend induction at 41 weeks for postdates, which is considered a medical indication.

Disclosure: The author has no commercial or financial conflicts of interest to disclose and no funding sources.
Division of Maternal-Fetal Medicine, Brigham and Women's Hospital, 75 Francis Street, Boston, MA 02115, USA
E-mail address: selittle@bwh.harvard.edu

Obstet Gynecol Clin N Am 44 (2017) 601–614
http://dx.doi.org/10.1016/j.ogc.2017.08.005
0889-8545/17/© 2017 Elsevier Inc. All rights reserved.

obgyn.theclinics.com

CURRENT TRENDS IN ELECTIVE INDUCTION

The overall rate of labor induction has increased dramatically in the United States over the last 30 years (**Fig. 1**). In 1990, less than 10% of deliveries were after an induced labor, increasing to 23% to 24% in 2005 before leveling off.[1,6-8] A similar trend has been seen in many other countries, across high, middle, and low income settings.[9] The increasing use of elective induction is driving the overall trend in labor induction rates. For example, among 6 US health care plans from 2001 to 2007, the overall rate of labor induction mirrored changes in the elective induction rate, which first increased from 11% to 14%, driving the overall rate from 28% to 32%, then declined back to 11% to bring the overall rate back down to 29%.[10]

IMPACT ON CESAREAN DELIVERY

One of the main concerns with labor induction is the potential impact it may have on cesarean delivery. Labor induction is often cited as a primary driver behind the increasing rate of cesarean delivery in the United States; cesarean delivery rates have increased nearly in parallel with increasing rates of labor induction.[8] It also makes intuitive sense to both patients and providers that induced labors would have a higher chance of ending in a cesarean delivery. However, the true relationship between labor induction and cesarean delivery is complex and, when analyzed more closely, it does not seem that labor induction is associated with a significantly increased risk of cesarean delivery.

The challenge with studying the effect of labor induction is in choosing the right comparison group. The comparison that is made most easily is between labors that are induced and those that are spontaneous; this is the comparison that providers see in the daily practice of obstetrics. When this comparison group is used, induced labors seem to be at approximately a 2-fold increased risk of cesarean delivery compared with spontaneous labors. For example, Heffner and colleagues[11] analyzed

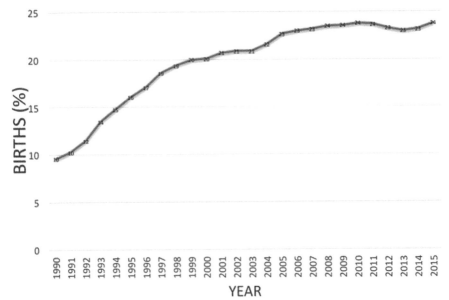

Fig. 1. Rates of labor induction in the United States from 1990 to 2015. (*Data from* Refs.[1,6-8])

more than 14,000 labors between 36 and 42 weeks of gestation. Labor induction was associated with a 1.7-fold increased risk of cesarean delivery in nulliparous women (95% confidence interval [CI], 1.48–1.95) and a 1.5-fold increased risk in multiparous women (95% CI, 1.1–2.0). Maslow and Sweeny[12] similarly found that, among 1135 low-risk, singleton vertex pregnancies at 38 to 41 weeks' gestation, elective labor induction was associated with 2.4-fold increased odds of cesarean delivery (95% CI, 1.2–4.9) in nulliparous women, independent of birthweight, maternal age, and gestational age, although there was no association in multiparous women.[12] Moreover, cervical examination status has been found to be a significant effect modifier in this relationship, with those women with an unfavorable cervix having the highest rates of cesarean delivery after labor induction.[13,14]

However, the problem is that women cannot choose to be in spontaneous labor at any given gestational age. The clinical choice is between immediate induction of labor or continued expectant management of pregnancy. During expectant management, spontaneous labor may occur (but at a later gestational age), a pregnancy complication may occur necessitating delivery (such as preeclampsia), or the pregnancy may reach postdates and labor may be induced at that time.

Retrospective studies that have recreated this expectant management of pregnancy comparison group have, in general, failed to find a significantly increased risk of cesarean delivery with labor induction. For example, Darney and colleagues[15] used California linked birth certificate and discharge data to recreate this comparison. They compared women who were electively induced (as per Joint Commission defined criteria from the International Classification of Diseases, Ninth Revision, billing codes) with women who were delivered at the next week of gestation or beyond. With this comparison, elective induction of labor was associated with reduced odds of cesarean delivery (eg, an adjusted odds ratio [aOR] of 0.46 at 39 weeks with a 95% CI of 0.41–0.52). Bailit and colleagues[16] similarly recreated this comparison group using Maternal-Fetal Medicine Units Network data to compare electively induced nulliparous women with those managed expectantly. At 38 and 40 weeks there was a slightly increased risk of cesarean delivery with labor induction (aOR, 1.5 and 1.3, respectively, both significant); however, at 39 weeks this increased risk was not significant (aOR, 1.13; 95% CI, 0.94–1.36). Gibson and colleagues[17] used data from the Safe Labor Consortium to compare elective induction with expectant management and found that labor induction was associated with a lower risk of cesarean delivery, and this held true regardless of parity or cervical examination status.

Recreating an expectant management retrospective cohort has inherent limitations. For one, many databases are done by week rather than day. Thus it is unclear whether women who delivered within the same week as the induction group should be included. Including them means that some women in the expectant management group may have delivered before the induction group, whereas omitting them leaves out women in the expectant management group who delivered several days after. Neither way is perfect, and several investigators have shown that the decision to include the same week or not in the expectant management group can lead to differing results.[18,19] Moreover, there is the potential for residual confounding with retrospective data, because the women who are induced may be fundamentally different from those managed expectantly.

The best data regarding the effect of labor induction come from randomized controlled trials in which the intervention was induction of labor. These trials have mainly been performed in populations with additional risk factors (eg, postdates, gestational diabetes, growth restriction, or advanced maternal age); nevertheless, the randomized nature of these trials provides the cleanest way to measure the

Table 1
Randomized controlled trials comparing induction of labor with expectant management

Study	Population	Design	Findings
Hannah et al, 1992[20]	Postterm pregnancies (≥41 wk) N = 3407	Induction of labor vs serial antenatal monitoring Induction via intracervical prostaglandin E2 (only included women with cervical dilatation <3 cm)	Cesarean delivery rate lower in induction group (21.2% vs 24.5%; P = .03)
Koopmans et al, 2009[21]	Gestational hypertension or mild preeclampsia (≥36 wk) N = 756	Induction at 36–41 wk with the diagnosis of gestational hypertension or mild preeclampsia compared with expectant management	Cesarean delivery rate lower in the induction group (14% vs 19%; nonsignificant)
Kjos et al, 1993[22]	Insulin-requiring gestational diabetes at 38 wk of gestation N = 200	Induction of labor within 5 d vs expectant management	Cesarean delivery rate lower in the induction group (25% vs 31%; nonsignificant)
Boers et al, 2010[23]	Suspected growth restriction (estimated fetal weight <10%) at ≥36 wk's gestation N = 650	Induction of labor at the time of diagnosis (≥36 wk) vs expectant management	Cesarean delivery rate lower in the expectant management group (13.7% vs 14.0%; nonsignificant)
Boulvain et al, 2015[24]	Suspected large-for-gestational-age fetuses (estimated fetal weight >95%) at 37 + 0 to 38 + 6 wk's gestation N = 822	Induction of labor within 3 d or diagnosis compared with expectant management	Cesarean delivery rate lower in the induction group (28% vs 32%; nonsignificant)
Walker et al, 2016[25]	Advanced maternal age (age ≥35 y) at 39 wk's gestation N = 619	Induction at 39 + 0 to 39 + 6 wk compared with expectant management	Cesarean delivery rates lower in the induction group (32% vs 33%; nonsignificant)
Amano et al, 1999[26]	Elective induction N = 194	Nulliparous women without medical complication, induction at 39 wk vs expectant management until 42 wk	Cesarean delivery rates lower in the expectant management group (5.6% vs 6.4%; nonsignificant)
Nielsen et al, 2005[27]	Elective induction, only included women with favorable cervix N = 226	Induction of labor at 39 wk vs expectant management until 42 wk	Cesarean delivery rates lower in the induction group (6.9% vs 7.3%; nonsignificant)
Miller et al, 2015[28]	Elective induction, nulliparous women with an unfavorable cervix N = 162	Induction of labor at 39 wk vs expectant management	Cesarean delivery rate lower in the expectant management group (17.7% vs 30.5%; nonsignificant)

independent effect of labor induction compared with expectant management. **Table 1** displays several of the key randomized trials. As shown, most of the trials found no significant difference in cesarean delivery rates between the two groups. Only 3 of the trials were in a healthy elective-induction population, and these were small trials, although they also failed to find a significant increase in cesarean delivery rates among women who were electively induced.

Several meta-analyses have been performed on these trials as well.[29-32] All the meta-analyses have found that labor induction is associated with significantly reduced odds of cesarean delivery compared with expectant management (aOR, 0.78–0.89). However, most of the trials in the meta-analyses were at 41 weeks or greater and/ or in higher-risk pregnancies. There are few trials at less than 41 weeks in an electively induced population.

IMPACT ON STILLBIRTH

One of the main reasons that many medically indicated inductions are recommended is for stillbirth prevention in populations with an increased risk of stillbirth. However, even in a low-risk population, stillbirths still occur at 39 or 40 weeks. Thus, elective induction at this gestation has the potential to avert this devastating pregnancy outcome.

Several researchers have analyzed whether policies limiting early term delivery (37 + 0 to 38 + 6 weeks) were associated with changes in term stillbirth rates (**Table 2**). Results have been mixed. Of the largest studies, Snowden and colleagues[33] found no difference in stillbirth rates in Oregon before and after policy changes limiting early elective delivery. Little and colleagues[34] found no difference in term stillbirth rates in the United States during a time period in which early elective delivery rates were decreasing. MacDorman and colleagues[35] also found no difference in the prospective risk of stillbirth by gestational age over a similar time period. However, Nicholson and colleagues[36] used slightly different data and methodology and did find a slight increase in stillbirth rates in the United States, likely as a consequence of changing practices with regard to early elective delivery.

Although the data thus far are reassuring that changes in delivery timing have not led to dramatic changes in term stillbirth rates, it still makes intuitive sense that elective delivery at 39 or 40 weeks would reduce the rate of stillbirth: stillbirths occur even in a healthy population at 39 or 40 weeks of gestation. However, given the low absolute risk of stillbirth, many elective inductions would have to be performed to prevent even 1 stillbirth. More research is needed on the absolute reduction in perinatal mortality that would be seen by a policy of routine elective induction after 39 weeks.

IMPACT ON NEONATAL AND MATERNAL MORBIDITY

There is a growing body of literature showing that early term delivery (37 + 0 to 38 + 6 weeks' gestation) is associated with an increased risk of neonatal morbidity compared with deliveries at 39 + 0 weeks or greater.[5,41] However, what about elective inductions after 39 weeks? The nadir of neonatal morbidity seems to be in the 39-week to 40-week range, with increasing neonatal complications occurring after 40 weeks and certainly after 41 weeks of gestation or beyond. However, elective induction is potentially associated with longer labors, which may also pose an increased risk for the neonate. Similarly, from the maternal standpoint, elective induction has the potential for benefit (eg, lower risk of macrosomia) but may be associated with increased morbidity from longer labor duration (eg, increased infection or hemorrhage).

Table 2
Term stillbirth rates after changes in elective delivery timing

Study	Setting/Intervention	Analysis	Finding
Ehrenthal et al, 2011[37]	Policy change limiting elective inductions before 39 wk at large regional academic center N = 24,028	Compared 2 y before change (2005–2006) with 2 y after change (2008–2009)	Increase in stillbirths at 37 and 38 wk (2.5–9.1 per 10,000; P = .032)
Oshiro et al, 2009[38]	9 urban medical centers within Intermountain Healthcare that participated in a process improvement program for reducing elective deliveries N = 28,150	Compared 2 y before the program (1999–2000) with 6 y after the program (2001–2006)	No change in the overall term stillbirth rate (0.15% before and 0.07% after; OR, 0.466; 95% CI, 0.33–0.65) or in the subgroups in the early term (37–38 wk)
Oshiro et al, 2013[39]	24 hospitals participating in the Big 5 State Prematurity Initiative, a quality improvement project to reduce elective early delivery N = 66,282	Compared outcomes across 4 quarters within 1 y	No change in the term stillbirth rate (1.1 per 1000 in the first quarter, 0.9 per 1000 in the last quarter) or in the subgroup in the early term (37–38 wk)
Little et al, 2014[40]	Practice changes to decrease early elective delivery at a single academic care center over a 5-y period (2006–2011) N = 21,343	Compared trends across the 5 y	No change in the term stillbirth rate (11.5 per 10,000 to 14.4 per 10,000; P = .55) or in the subgroup in the early term (37–38 wk)
Little et al, 2015[34]	Analysis of birth certificate and fetal death data from United States from 2005–2011 when early term delivery rates declined N ~ 25 million	Analyzed state-level trends in term stillbirth	No change in the overall term stillbirth rate (123 per 100,000 in 2005 to 130 per 100,000 in 2011; P = .189) nor any correlation between state-level reduction in early term delivery and state-level change in term stillbirth

MacDorman et al, 2015[35]	Analysis of gestational age–specific prospective risk of stillbirth from fetal death and birth certificate data in the United States from 2006 to 2012 N ~25 million	Analyzed the prospective risk of stillbirth at each gestational age and whether this changed over time	No difference in the prospective risk of stillbirth from 21–42 wk of gestation from 2006 to 2012
Nicholson et al, 2016[36]	Analysis of state-level data from 46 states from 2007 to 2013 N ~25 million	Term stillbirth rates from 2007–2009 compared with rates from 2011–2013	Term stillbirth rate increased from 1.103 per 1000 in 2007–2009 to 1.177 per 1000 in 2011–2013 (RR, 1.067; 95% CI, 1.038–1.096)
Snowden et al, 2016[33]	Term and postterm, nonanomalous, singleton births in Oregon after a hard stop on early term elective delivery N = 181,034	Stillbirth rates compared before (2008–2010) and after (2012–2013) the hard stop	No change in stillbirth rates between before (0.10%) and after (0.12%) the change (aOR 1.20; 95% CI, 0.88–1.63)

Abbreviations: OR, odds ratio; RR, relative risk.

Similar to analyzing the impact of induction on cesarean delivery, the correct comparison group for analyzing maternal and neonatal morbidity is an expectant management cohort. Several studies have recreated this comparison group (**Table 3**). For maternal outcomes, elective induction at 39 or 40 weeks seems to be associated with a lower rate of infection, hemorrhage, and severe perineal lacerations. For neonatal outcomes, there seems to be an overall reduction in morbidity, although the findings were not consistent across all studies, with 1 study finding an increased rate of neonatal intensive care unit (NICU) admission after elective induction at 39 or 40 weeks.[19] Others have also noted a decreased risk of meconium-stained fluid with induction before 41 weeks compared with expectant management.[42]

The randomized controlled trial data comparing labor induction with expectant management is less informative for neonatal/maternal morbidities given that most trials occurred in high-risk groups (eg, fetal growth restriction or maternal hypertension) in which baseline risks of maternal/neonatal morbidity are likely to be significantly different from an elective induction cohort. However, the study in women of advanced maternal age provides some information.[25] This study was a randomized trial of induction of labor at 39 weeks in women who were 35 years of age or older and included 619 women. The expectant management group was delivered, on average, a week after the induction group. There was no significant difference in maternal outcomes (eg, infection, postpartum hemorrhage, or shoulder dystocia) or in neonatal outcomes (eg, cord gas, need for intervention, or NICU admission) with induction at 39 weeks.

Overall, it seems that elective induction after 39 weeks may be associated with a reduction in some maternal/neonatal morbidities in retrospective data. However, there is a need for more prospective/randomized data to confirm these findings.

IMPACT ON PATIENT EXPERIENCE AND COST

Even if elective induction is associated with lower rates of morbidity and mortality, the absolute rate of complication in a healthy singleton cohort between 39 and 41 weeks is low. Thus, the impact that elective induction has on patient experience and cost/resource use must also be considered.

The Listening to Mothers surveys report high rates of intervention in labor on even healthy pregnancies and mothers report feeling a lack of control or pressure to accept these interventions.[43,44] Shetty and colleagues[45] report that women who spontaneously labor report overall higher rates of satisfaction with their labor experiences. More research is needed on the psychosocial impact that elective labor induction has on women. Labor induction has also been associated with decreased rates of breastfeeding compared with spontaneous labor.[46]

Moreover, labor induction is more costly than spontaneous labor.[12,47,48] However, this does not take into account that not all women managed expectantly labor spontaneously, or that expectant management leads to additional costs (eg, antenatal testing and prenatal visits). The cost relationship is more complex when these factors are taken into account, and the true relationship between cost and elective induction is not clear.[49] A cost-effectiveness model at 41 weeks found that a policy of routine labor induction at this gestational age was slightly more expensive but led to improved outcomes and was within a cost-effective range.[50] However, it may not be possible to generalize this finding to lower gestational ages. An economic evaluation of the randomized controlled trial of elective induction at 39 weeks for women of advanced maternal age found that induction of labor in this cohort produced slight cost savings,[51] but it is not clear whether this can be generalized to a lower-risk cohort with likely less need for antenatal surveillance.

Table 3
Impact of elective induction after 39 weeks on maternal and neonatal risks/benefits

Study	Design	Maternal Risks/Benefits	Neonatal Risks/Benefits
Gibson et al, 2014[17]	Safe Labor Consortium data (19 hospitals) Elective induction vs expectant management N = 131,243	Nulliparas: No difference in bleeding complications, ICU admissions, third-degree/fourth-degree lacerations, shoulder dystocias Decrease in infections: aOR 39 wk: 0.41 (0.33–0.50) aOR 40 wk: 0.45 (0.38–0.55) Multiparas: No difference in bleeding complications, ICU admissions, shoulder dystocias Decrease in infections: aOR 39 wk: 0.34 (0.25–0.47) aOR 40 wk: Nonsignificant Decrease in third-degree/fourth-degree lacerations: aOR 39 wk: 0.61 (0.49–0.76) aOR 40 wk: 0.67 (0.46–0.98)	Nulliparas: No difference in perinatal death Decrease in composite morbidity[a]: aOR 39 wk: 0.75 (0.61–0.92) aOR 40 wk: 0.65 (0.54–0.80) Decrease in composite respiratory morbidity[b]: aOR 39 wk: 0.54 (0.37–0.78) aOR 40 wk: 0.59 (0.42–0.82) Multiparas: No difference in perinatal death Decrease in composite morbidity[a]: aOR 39 wk: 0.59 (0.49–0.71) aOR 40 wk: Not significant Decrease in composite respiratory morbidity[b]: aOR 39 wk: 0.57 (0.42–0.78) aOR 40 wk: Not significant

(continued on next page)

Table 3
(continued)

Study	Design	Maternal Risks/Benefits	Neonatal Risks/Benefits
Darney et al, 2013[15]	California linked birth certificate and hospital discharge data Elective induction vs expectant management N = 362, 154	Decrease in third-degree/fourth-degree lacerations: aOR 39 wk: 0.65 (0.55–0.78) aOR 40 wk: 0.82 (0.68–1.00)	No change in hyperbilirubinemia or shoulder dystocia Decrease in NICU admission: aOR at 39 wk: 0.68 (0.59–0.78) aOR at 40 wk: 0.70 (0.59–0.83) Decrease in respiratory distress: aOR 39 wk: 0.59 (0.46–0.76) aOR 40 wk: 0.47 (0.34–0.65) Decrease in macrosomia: aOR 39 wk: 0.97 (0.72–0.87) aOR 40 wk: not significant
Stock et al, 2012[19]	Scottish birth records Elective induction vs expectant management N = 1,271,549	Decrease in postpartum hemorrhage: aOR 39 wk: 0.90 (0.83–0.98) aOR 40 wk: 0.82 (0.77–0.86) Decrease in anal sphincter injury: aOR 39 wk: 0.62 (0.43–0.89) aOR 40 wk: 0.74 (0.60–0.91)	Increase in NICU admission: aOR 39 wk: 1.17 (1.07–1.26) aOR 40 wk: 1.14 (1.09–1.20)

Abbreviations: HIE, hypoxic-ischemic encephalopathy; ICU, intensive care unit; IVH, intraventricular hemorrhage; NICU, neonatal intensive care unit; PNA, pneumonia; PPV, positive pressure ventilation; RDS, respiratory distress syndrome; TTN, transient tachypnea of the newborn.
[a] Includes birth injury, sepsis, PNA, IVH, aspiration, HIE, RDS, seizures, oliguria, myocardial injury, ventilator use, continuous PPV, TTN, transfusions, or surfactant use.
[b] Includes O$_2$ use, continuous PPV, TTN, or surfactant administration.

In summary, although a labor induction is clearly more costly than spontaneous labor, there is not enough information at this time to say whether elective induction is more costly, when the appropriate comparison (expectant management) and the resultant differences in outpatient costs, as well as any potential differences in health outcomes, are considered.

SUMMARY

Elective induction of labor is increasingly common in the United States. When using the correct comparison group (women expectantly managed at a given gestational age and beyond) it seems that elective induction of labor is not associated with significantly increased risks, and may be associated with lower rates of cesarean delivery and improved maternal and neonatal morbidity. There is also the potential to decrease the stillbirth rate, although studies have thus far failed to find significant changes in term stillbirth after changes in delivery timing at term. Nevertheless, the potential benefits of elective induction must be weighed against the potential for decreased patient satisfaction, overmedicalization of the labor process, and the impact on breastfeeding and cost/resource use. Further prospective studies are needed to better assess the full impact of elective induction on maternal and neonatal morbidity, maternal well-being, and cost.

REFERENCES

1. Martin JA, Hamilton BE, Osterman MJK, et al. Births: final data for 2015. Natl Vital Stat Rep 2017;66(1):1.
2. Berghella V, Blackwell SC, Ramin SM, et al. Use and misuse of the term "elective" in obstetrics. Obstet Gynecol 2011;117(2 Pt 1):372–6.
3. American College of Obstetricians and Gynecologists. ACOG committee opinion no. 561: nonmedically indicated early-term deliveries. Obstet Gynecol 2013; 121(4):911–5.
4. Darney BG, Caughey AB. Elective induction of labor symposium: nomenclature, research methodological issues, and outcomes. Clin Obstet Gynecol 2014;57(2): 343–62.
5. Tita ATN, Landon MB, Spong CY, et al. Timing of elective repeat cesarean delivery at term and neonatal outcomes. N Engl J Med 2009;360(2):111–20.
6. Martin JA, Hamilton BE, Osterman MJ, et al. Births: final data for 2013. Natl Vital Stat Rep 2015;64(1):1–65.
7. Hamilton BE, Martin JA, Osterman MJK, et al. Births: final data for 2014. Natl Vital Stat Rep 2015;64(12):1–64.
8. Osterman MJK, Martin JA. Recent declines in induction of labor by gestational age. NCHS Data Brief 2014;(155):1–8.
9. Vogel JP, Gülmezoglu AMM, Hofmeyr GJ, et al. Global perspectives on elective induction of labor. Clin Obstet Gynecol 2014;57(2):331–42.
10. Dublin S, Johnson KE, Walker RL, et al. Trends in elective labor induction for six United States health plans, 2001-2007. J Womens Health (Larchmt) 2014;23(11): 904–11.
11. Heffner LJ, Elkin E, Fretts RC. Impact of labor induction, gestational age, and maternal age on cesarean delivery rates. Obstet Gynecol 2003;102(2):287–93.
12. Maslow AS, Sweeny AL. Elective induction of labor as a risk factor for cesarean delivery among low-risk women at term. Obstet Gynecol 2000;95(6 Pt 1):917–22.

13. Johnson DP, Davis NR, Brown AJ. Risk of cesarean delivery after induction at term in nulliparous women with an unfavorable cervix. Am J Obstet Gynecol 2003;188(6):1565–9 [discussion: 1569–72].

14. Vrouenraets FPJM, Roumen FJME, Dehing CJG, et al. Bishop score and risk of cesarean delivery after induction of labor in nulliparous women. Obstet Gynecol 2005;105(4):690–7.

15. Darney BG, Snowden JM, Cheng YW, et al. Elective induction of labor at term compared with expectant management. Obstet Gynecol 2013;122(4):761–9.

16. Bailit JL, Grobman W, Zhao Y, et al. Nonmedically indicated induction vs expectant treatment in term nulliparous women. Am J Obstet Gynecol 2015;212(1): 103.e1–7.

17. Gibson KS, Waters TP, Bailit JL. Maternal and neonatal outcomes in electively induced low-risk term pregnancies. Am J Obstet Gynecol 2014;211(3): 249.e1–16.

18. Glantz JC. Term labor induction compared with expectant management. Obstet Gynecol 2010;115(1):70–6.

19. Stock SJ, Ferguson E, Duffy A, et al. Outcomes of elective induction of labour compared with expectant management: population based study. BMJ 2012; 344:e2838.

20. Hannah ME, Hannah WJ, Hellmann J, et al. Induction of labor as compared with serial antenatal monitoring in post-term pregnancy. A randomized controlled trial. The Canadian Multicenter Post-term Pregnancy Trial Group. N Engl J Med 1992; 326(24):1587–92.

21. Koopmans CM, Bijlenga D, Groen H, et al. Induction of labour versus expectant monitoring for gestational hypertension or mild pre-eclampsia after 36 weeks' gestation (HYPITAT): a multicentre, open-label randomised controlled trial. Lancet 2009;374(9694):979–88.

22. Kjos SL, Henry OA, Montoro M, et al. Insulin-requiring diabetes in pregnancy: a randomized trial of active induction of labor and expectant management. Am J Obstet Gynecol 1993;169(3):611–5.

23. Boers KE, Vijgen SMC, Bijlenga D, et al. Induction versus expectant monitoring for intrauterine growth restriction at term: randomised equivalence trial (DIGITAT). BMJ 2010;341:c7087.

24. Boulvain M, Senat M-V, Perrotin F, et al. Induction of labour versus expectant management for large-for-date fetuses: a randomised controlled trial. Lancet 2015;385(9987):2600–5.

25. Walker KF, Bugg GJ, Macpherson M, et al. Randomized trial of labor induction in women 35 years of age or older. N Engl J Med 2016;374(9):813–22.

26. Amano K, Saito K, Shoda T, et al. Elective induction of labor at 39 weeks of gestation: a prospective randomized trial. J Obstet Gynaecol Res 1999;25(1):33–7.

27. Nielsen PE, Howard BC, Hill CC, et al. Comparison of elective induction of labor with favorable Bishop scores versus expectant management: a randomized clinical trial. J Matern Fetal Neonatal Med 2005;18(1):59–64.

28. Miller NR, Cypher RL, Foglia LM, et al. Elective induction of labor compared with expectant management of nulliparous women at 39 weeks of gestation: a randomized controlled trial. Obstet Gynecol 2015;126(6):1258–64.

29. Wood S, Cooper S, Ross S. Does induction of labour increase the risk of caesarean section? A systematic review and meta-analysis of trials in women with intact membranes. BJOG 2014;121(6):674–85 [discussion: 685].

30. Mishanina E, Rogozinska E, Thatthi T, et al. Use of labour induction and risk of cesarean delivery: a systematic review and meta-analysis. CMAJ 2014;186(9): 665–73.

31. Caughey AB, Sundaram V, Kaimal AJ, et al. Systematic review: elective induction of labor versus expectant management of pregnancy. Ann Intern Med 2009; 151(4):252–63. W53–63.

32. Gülmezoglu AM, Crowther CA, Middleton P, et al. Induction of labour for improving birth outcomes for women at or beyond term. Cochrane Database Syst Rev 2012;(6):CD004945.

33. Snowden JM, Muoto I, Darney BG, et al. Oregon's hard-stop policy limiting elective early-term deliveries: association with obstetric procedure use and health outcomes. Obstet Gynecol 2016;128(6):1389–96.

34. Little SE, Zera CA, Clapp MA, et al. A multi-state analysis of early-term delivery trends and the association with term stillbirth. Obstet Gynecol 2015;126(6): 1138–45.

35. MacDorman MF, Reddy UM, Silver RM. Trends in stillbirth by gestational age in the United States, 2006–2012. Obstet Gynecol 2015;126(6):1146–50.

36. Nicholson JM, Kellar LC, Ahmad S, et al. US term stillbirth rates and the 39-week rule: a cause for concern? Am J Obstet Gynecol 2016;214(5):621.e1-9.

37. Ehrenthal DB, Hoffman MK, Jiang X, et al. Neonatal outcomes after implementation of guidelines limiting elective delivery before 39 weeks of gestation. Obstet Gynecol 2011;118(5):1047–55.

38. Oshiro BT, Henry E, Wilson J, et al, Women and Newborn Clinical Integration Program. Decreasing elective deliveries before 39 weeks of gestation in an integrated health care system. Obstet Gynecol 2009;113(4):804–11.

39. Oshiro BT, Kowalewski L, Sappenfield W, et al. A multistate quality improvement program to decrease elective deliveries before 39 weeks of gestation. Obstet Gynecol 2013;121(5):1025–31.

40. Little SE, Robinson JN, Puopolo KM, et al. The effect of obstetric practice change to reduce early term delivery on perinatal outcome. J Perinatol 2014;34(3): 176–80.

41. Chiossi G, Lai Y, Landon MB, et al. Timing of delivery and adverse outcomes in term singleton repeat cesarean deliveries. Obstet Gynecol 2013;121(3):561–9.

42. Caughey AB, Sundaram V, Kaimal AJ, et al. Maternal and neonatal outcomes of elective induction of labor. Evid Rep Technol Assess (Full Rep) 2009;176:1–257.

43. Sakala C, Declercq ER, Corry MP. Listening to mothers: the first national U.S. survey of women's childbearing experiences. J Obstet Gynecol Neonatal Nurs 2002; 31(6):633–4.

44. Declercq ER, Sakala C, Corry MP, et al. Major survey findings of listening to mothers(SM) III: pregnancy and birth: report of the Third National U.S. Survey of Women's Childbearing Experiences. J Perinat Educ 2014;23(1):9.

45. Shetty A, Burt R, Rice P, et al. Women's perceptions, expectations and satisfaction with induced labour–a questionnaire-based study. Eur J Obstet Gynecol Reprod Biol 2005;123(1):56–61.

46. Zanardo V, Bertin M, Sansone L, et al. The adaptive psychological changes of elective induction of labor in breastfeeding women. Early Hum Dev 2017;104: 13–6.

47. Allen VM, O'Connell CM, Farrell SA, et al. Economic implications of method of delivery. Am J Obstet Gynecol 2005;193(1):192–7.

48. Garcia-Simon R, Montañes A, Clemente J, et al. Economic implications of labor induction. Int J Gynaecol Obstet 2016;133(1):112–5.

49. Grobman WA. Costs of elective induction of labor. Clin Obstet Gynecol 2014; 57(2):363–8.

50. Kaimal AJ, Little SE, Odibo AO, et al. Cost-effectiveness of elective induction of labor at 41 weeks in nulliparous women. Am J Obstet Gynecol 2011;204(2): 137.e1-9.

51. Walker KF, Dritsaki M, Bugg G, et al. Labour induction near term for women aged 35 or over: an economic evaluation. BJOG 2017;124(6):929–34.

Update on Fetal Monitoring
Overview of Approaches and Management of Category II Tracings

Nandini Raghuraman, MD, MS*, Alison G. Cahill, MD, MSCI

KEYWORDS

- Category II • Intrauterine resuscitation • Electronic fetal monitoring • Management

KEY POINTS

- Nonreassuring fetal heart tracings (FHTs) account for a significant portion of unplanned cesarean deliveries in the United States.
- Category II FHTs encompass a broad range of fetal heart rate patterns, some of which are better predictors of neonatal acidemia than others.
- Adjunct intrapartum tests of fetal well-being may help triage those with category II FHTs.
- Intrauterine resuscitation techniques should target the underlying etiology of uteroplacental insufficiency or cord compression.

INTRODUCTION

Electronic fetal monitoring (EFM) is widely used for assessment of intrapartum fetal status and has become integral to labor management. More than 80% of laboring patients in the United States have intrapartum EFM.[1] Intrapartum fetal assessment has largely evolved over the past few decades from its inception as intermittent auscultation to its progression to fetal scalp sampling and now, EFM. Nonreassuring fetal status as interpreted on the basis of EFM accounts for nearly a quarter of primary cesarean deliveries.[2] Thus, as an engrained component of modern-day obstetric practice, EFM requires a careful understanding of its strengths, limitations, and management.

Disclosure Statement: The authors do not have any commercial or financial conflicts of interest.
Department of Obstetrics and Gynecology, Division of Maternal-Fetal Medicine, Washington University School of Medicine in St. Louis, 660 South Euclid Avenue, Maternity Building, 5th Floor, St Louis, MO 63110, USA
* Corresponding author.
E-mail address: raghuramann@wudosis.wustl.edu

Obstet Gynecol Clin N Am 44 (2017) 615–624
http://dx.doi.org/10.1016/j.ogc.2017.08.007
0889-8545/17/© 2017 Elsevier Inc. All rights reserved.

IS ELECTRONIC FETAL MONITORING PREDICTIVE OF NEONATAL OUTCOMES?

Fetal heart tracings (FHTs) are a reflection of the fetal central nervous system response to intrauterine hypoxia. The theorized benefit of EFM is to identify and intervene on fetal hypoxia and/or acidosis, thereby reducing adverse neonatal outcomes. Results of studies evaluating EFM's role in preventing adverse neonatal outcomes are mixed, however, at best.

EFM has been compared with intermittent auscultation in several prospective studies and reviews. Although a reduction in neurologic outcomes has not been shown, there is evidence to suggest reduction in perinatal mortality, in particular intrapartum death.[1,3–5] In their observational study of a national birth cohort, Chen and colleagues[1] found that intrapartum EFM was associated with lower early neonatal and infant mortality. Additionally, the investigators observed a significantly lower rate of neonatal seizures in those with intrapartum continuous EFM, a finding similar to that seen in a Cochrane review of 13 trials comparing EFM to intermittent auscultation.[6] Despite seeing a difference in neonatal seizures, the Cochrane review found no difference in perinatal mortality or neurodevelopmental outcomes, including hypoxic ischemic encephalopathy and cerebral palsy.[6] A consistent finding among many of these studies is the observed increased risk of operative vaginal delivery and cesarean section with continuous EFM.[1,3,5–7]

ELECTRONIC FETAL MONITORING PATTERNS AND CLASSIFICATION

The widespread use of EFM, despite lack of consistent proof of benefit, rests on the notion of detecting and intervening on signs of fetal acidemia. In their comparison of continuous intrapartum EFM to intermittent auscultation, Vintzileos and colleagues[8] concluded that EFM had higher sensitivity and positive predictive value in detecting fetal acidemia at birth. Recent evidence, however, suggests that EFM with algorithm-assisted interpretation identifies only half of infants born with metabolic acidemia.[9]

The Eunice Kennedy Shriver National Institute of Child Health and Human Development (NICHD) classification of FHT in 2008[10] standardized EFM language by creating 3 categories based on fetal heart rate baseline, variability, accelerations, and subtypes of decelerations, with category III FHT having the strongest association with abnormal fetal acid-base status (**Box 1**). The American College of Obstetricians and Gynecologists (ACOG) recommends using this 3-tiered nomenclature system for intrapartum EFM interpretation.[11] Despite moderate interobserver reliability at best[12] the NICHD system remains the mainstay of EFM management throughout the United States.

Certain patterns of EFM decelerations or variability are associated with adverse neonatal outcomes. A 2012 retrospective cohort study of more than 5000 patients undergoing intrapartum EFM identified features of EFM, in particular deceleration frequency and severity, which were predictive of acidemia independent of the NICHD categories. Within the NICHD-defined EFM features, repetitive prolonged decelerations, tachycardia, recurrent variable decelerations, and recurrent late decelerations were identified as predictors of acidemia.[13]

Variability in fetal heart rate baseline also seems to play a key role in the prediction of neonatal acidemia. Minimal variability has been shown to correlate with neonatal acidemia but with positive predictive values as low as 18%.[14,15] Moderate variability, however, seems protective of acidemia as demonstrated by Williams and Galerneau[15] in a study showing that a majority of patients with moderate variability and accelerations, even in the presence of late or variable decelerations, had umbilical artery pH greater

---

Box 1
National Institute of Child Health and Human Development 3-tiered fetal heart rate interpretation system

Category I

Predictive of normal fetal acid-base status

Routine intrapartum care

All of the following
Baseline 110 bpm to 160 bpm
Moderate FHR variability
No late or variable decelerations
± Early decelerations
± Accelerations

Category II

Indeterminate

Evaluate, consider intrauterine resuscitation, continued surveillance

Any of the following
Baseline <110 bpm without absent baseline variability
Baseline >160 bpm
Minimal FHR variability
Absent FHR variability without recurrent decelerations
Marked FHR variability
Absence of accelerations after fetal stimulation
Recurrent variable decelerations with minimal or moderate FHR variability
Prolonged deceleration ≥2 minutes but <10 minutes
Recurrent late decelerations with moderate FHR variability
Variable decelerations with other characteristics, such as slow return to baseline, overshoots, or shoulders

Category III

Predictive of abnormal fetal acid-base status

Prompt evaluation, intrauterine resuscitation, expedite delivery if no improvement with resuscitation

Any of the following
Absent FHR variability AND recurrent late decelerations OR recurrent variable decelerations OR bradycardia
Sinusoidal pattern

Abbreviation: FHR, fetal heart rate.
Adapted from Macones GA, Hankins GD, Spong CY, et al. The 2008 National Institute of Child Health and Human Development workshop report on electronic fetal monitoring: update on definitions, interpretation, and research guidelines. Obstet Gynecol 2008;112(3):664; with permission.

---

than 7.0. Future studies in EFM should further address the relationship between specific FHT patterns and adverse neonatal outcomes.

MANAGEMENT OF CATEGORY II FETAL HEART TRACINGS
Adjunct Tests of Fetal Well-Being

The majority of intrapartum FHT is category II.[16] In this indeterminate category and in the case of category III FHT, additional tests of fetal well-being can be helpful in guiding further management. In the presence of minimal or absent variability, a digital fetal scalp stimulation may be performed if the cervix is dilated. A fetal acceleration in response to the scalp stimulation is highly predictive of fetal pH greater than 7.20.[17,18] Alternatively, if the cervix is closed, vibroacoustic stimulation on the maternal abdomen may be considered.[19]

Historically, fetal scalp sampling was a commonly used intrapartum ancillary test for fetal assessment. Fetal scalp sampling involved puncture of the fetal scalp to obtain capillary blood analysis of fetal pH and lactate as a secondary assessment of fetal well-being in the setting of abnormal FHT. The addition of fetal scalp sampling to EFM, however, did not yield improved predictive value for adverse neonatal outcomes nor did it reduce the risk of operative intervention.[6,20] Experts determined that factors, such as amniotic fluid, contamination of the sample with air, and sampling from a peripheral site affected by fetal vasoconstriction contributed to the limited predictive value of fetal scalp sampling.[20,21] The practical difficulties involved in this approach, including the need for well-maintained equipment, invasive technique, trained personnel, technical competence, and unreliable results, led to the eventual demise of this practice in the Unites States.[22]

Fetal pulse oximetry was an additional adjunct test of intrapartum fetal status that has fallen out of favor. It was originally designed as an intrapartum tool for real-time measurement of fetal arterial oxygen saturation by determining the ratio of oxyhemoglobin to deoxyhemoglobin using wavelength assessment.[23] The noninvasive technique of sensor placement, compared with fetal scalp sampling, made this form of monitoring appealing. A large, multicenter randomized controlled trial performed by the NICHD comparing masked to unmasked oximeter results concluded that physician knowledge of intrapartum fetal oxygen saturation had no significant effect on the rates of cesarean delivery or neonatal outcomes.[24] Subsequently, the Food and Drug Administration did not approve its use after several other randomized trials and reviews found no difference in cesarean delivery rates or neonatal outcomes with the use of fetal pulse oximetry compared with EFM alone.[24,25]

Recently, fetal ST segment waveform analysis (STAN) has been proposed as an adjunct test for detection of intrapartum fetal hypoxemia. In this form of monitoring, a fetal scalp electrode (FSE) is used to obtain a fetal ECG. Analysis of the ST segment and T waves then provides information about myocardial changes and metabolic status. A recent large Maternal-Fetal Medicine Units Network trial of more than 11,000 patients, however, showed no reduction in the composite outcome of intrapartum fetal death, neonatal death, Apgar score less than 3 at 5 minutes, neonatal seizure, umbilical artery pH less than 7.05 with base deficit greater than 12 mmol/L, neonatal intubation, or neonatal encephalopathy. There was also no difference in cesarean delivery or operative delivery rates between groups.[26] A subsequent systematic review and meta-analysis of 7 trials concluded that use of STAN made no difference in cesarean delivery rates or neonatal outcomes.[27]

Intrauterine pressure catheters (IUPCs) and FSEs are commonly used intrapartum devices for monitoring contractions and fetal status. FSE placement allows for improved tracking of FHT that may otherwise be discontinuous or unreliable transabdominally (ie, maternal morbid obesity). Similarly, IUPC placement allows for assessment of contraction adequacy, amnioinfusion, and improved tocometry fidelity in patients who are difficult to monitor transabdominally. In a retrospective cohort study by Harper and colleagues,[28] patients with an IUPC had a 2-fold increased risk of intrapartum or postpartum fever and were more likely to have a cesarean delivery compared with those without internal monitors. This relationship may be affected by the underlying indication for IUPC placement. The use of FSE alone was associated with a decrease in the risk of cesarean delivery with no associated increase in fever. A recent retrospective cohort study by Kawakita and colleagues[29] evaluated the risk of neonatal complications with FSE placement. The investigators found a low but statistically significant risk of neonatal morbidity in the form of scalp injury and cephalohematoma with FSE placement. These studies highlight the potential safety risks associated with internal monitor use and suggest avoiding routine use of internal monitors unless clinically indicated.

In Utero Resuscitation

The presence of category II FHT calls for a careful assessment of factors that may be contributing to fetal hypo-oxygenation. These factors then guide choice of intrauterine resuscitation technique (**Table 1**). Recurrent variable decelerations represent umbilical cord compression. Amnioinfusion is a resuscitation technique aimed at alleviating cord compression by infusion of normal saline into the uterus via an IUPC. Several studies have demonstrated benefit of amnioinfusion in alleviating recurrent variable decelerations and reducing cesarean deliveries for nonreassuring fetal status, with no associated infection risk.[30–34]

In the presence of recurrent late or variable decelerations, maternal repositioning, particularly to the left lateral recumbent position, may improve uteroplacental perfusion and release umbilical cord compression. Carbonne and colleagues[35] studied the effects of various maternal positions during labor on fetal pulse oximetry readings and found that the maternal supine position was associated with a lower fetal oxygen saturation than the left lateral position. This difference in fetal oxygen saturation was attributed to aortic compression by the gravid uterus. The study population was limited, however, to those with normal FHT. There remain few to no data on the effect of maternal position change for category II FHT on neonatal outcomes. Uterine tachysystole, defined as greater than 5 contractions in 10 minutes over an average of 30 minutes, is associated with abnormal FHT due to shortened uterine relaxation time.[36,37] Administration of terbutaline and/or discontinuation of oxytocin may be considered in the setting of tachysystole and associated nonreassuring fetal tracings.

Intrapartum maternal oxygen administration is often performed for FHTs that are thought to reflect fetal hypoxia, such as recurrent late decelerations or prolonged decelerations. The theoretic benefit of such oxygen administration is to increase oxygen delivery to the fetus, thereby reversing hypoxemia and resultant acidemia. Although

Table 1
Intrauterine resuscitation techniques

Intervention	Potential Benefit
Maternal lateral repositioning	• Avoids compression of maternal great vessels and improves uteroplacental perfusion • Alleviates umbilical cord compression
Reduction or discontinuation of oxytocin Administration of tocolytic	• Reduces uterine tachysystole and subsequent fetal hypo-oxygenation
Maternal oxygen administration	• Increases oxygen transfer to fetal umbilical vein
Intravenous fluid bolus	• Improves maternal hypovolemia and increases uteroplacental perfusion
Amnioinfusion	• Alleviates umbilical cord compression and recurrent variable decelerations

Adapted from American College of Obstetricians and Gynecologists. Practice Bulletin no. 116: management of intrapartum fetal heart rate tracings. Obstet Gynecol 2010;116(5):1232–40; with permission.

studies have shown increased umbilical vein oxygen content and resolution of fetal heart rate decelerations with oxygen administration,[38–41] there is no evidence that this practice improves neonatal outcomes. A recent observational study demonstrated an increased risk of neonatal morbidity in the setting of intrauterine hyperoxemia and acidemia.[42] The risks of free radical damage with prolonged oxygen exposure should also be considered.[43]

Collectively, there is limited evidence that the intrauterine resuscitation techniques recommended by ACOG[44] improve neonatal outcomes. In the absence of high-quality evidence demonstrating benefit of these techniques, providers should identify the etiology of perceived fetal hypoxia and select a resuscitation method most appropriate for the cause. Future research should address the risks and benefits of these methods either individually or in combination as bundled intrauterine resuscitative care.

INTRAPARTUM FACTORS TO CONSIDER
Neuraxial Anesthesia

Up to 10% of patients with epidural or combined spinal-epidural analgesia may experience associated hypotension.[45] Maternal hypotension in this setting can lead to uteroplacental hypoperfusion and subsequent changes in FHT that reflect fetal hypoxia. Another proposed mechanism for category II FHT after neuraxial anesthesia administration is sudden-onset imbalance of maternal adrenaline and noradrenaline that results in uterine hypertonia.[46–48] A recent systematic review and meta-analysis by Hattler and colleagues[49] showed that combined spinal-epidural anesthesia was associated with a higher risk of fetal bradycardia and nonreassuring FHT than epidural anesthesia, although nonreassuring FHT was not well defined. Similar observational studies have also demonstrated FHT abnormalities in association with intrathecal opioid administration.[50,51]

Continuous EFM at time of and after neuraxial anesthesia administration should be considered so that providers may intervene for associated FHT changes. Such interventions may include intravenous fluid hydration and/or administration of phenylephrine or ephedrine for maternal hypotension.

Magnesium

Magnesium sulfate, a commonly administered medication for tocolysis, eclampsia prevention, or fetal neuroprotection, crosses the placenta with detectable levels in the neonate.[52] Several observational studies have shown a decrease in fetal heart rate baseline and variability during magnesium exposure.[52–54] A randomized controlled trial of magnesium sulfate versus sodium chloride infusion in nonlaboring patients demonstrated a decrease in fetal heart rate baseline and variability after 3 hours of magnesium infusion.[55] The clinical utility of these findings may be limited, however, given the small 2 beats per minute (bpm) change in baseline that was observed. Another trial by Twickler and colleagues[56] found a decrease in baseline as high as 10 bpm to 12 bpm with magnesium administration.

Intrauterine Growth Restriction

Chronic placental insufficiency and subsequent intrauterine growth restriction (IUGR) may be associated with a delay in fetal central nervous system maturation that subsequently has an impact on FHTs. An observational study of 24 nonlaboring patients with IUGR matched to patients with normally grown fetuses demonstrated fewer accelerations in the IUGR group.[57] Similarly, in a case control study by Vinkesteijn and colleagues,[58] patients with IUGR were found to have reduced fetal heart rate variability. These findings may not be applicable to intrapartum FHT associated with IUGR. Epplin and colleagues[59] studied second-stage fetal heart rate patterns in patients with IUGR and found that IUGR fetuses were less likely to have accelerations and were more likely to have late decelerations compared with those that were normally grown. There was no difference in bradycardia or variability between groups. Underlying placental insufficiency and associated changes in fetal systemic regulation may predispose patients with IUGR to category II FHT in labor. The efficacy of intrauterine resuscitation techniques in this setting remains unanswered.

Meconium

Meconium stained fluid is found in 12% of all deliveries and in more than 20% of patients with category II FHT.[60] Meconium in association with category II FHT significantly increases the risk of neonatal morbidity even after excluding neonates diagnosed with meconium aspiration syndrome. Furthermore, this risk is significantly increased in the presence of thick, rather than thin, meconium.[60] Specific FHT patterns within the broader group of category II FHT that are associated with neonatal morbidity in the presence of meconium include prolonged decelerations, severe variable decelerations, bradycardia and tachycardia.[61] The presence or absence of meconium allows for risk stratification among patients with category II FHT. Observational studies and randomized controlled trials evaluating the utility of amnioinfusion for prevention of meconium-related neonatal morbidity have produced mixed results and the benefit of amnioinfusion for the combination of meconium and category II FHT remains unclear.[31,62,63]

SUMMARY

Category II FHT encompasses a broad range of fetal heart rate patterns and is indeterminate in its ability to predict fetal acidemia. Deceleration frequency, deceleration severity, and variability, however, may be key components within category II FHT that predict adverse neonatal outcomes. Intrauterine resuscitation techniques should be selected and administered based on the suspected etiology of fetal hypoxia (maternal hypotension, cord compression, and so forth). Clinical factors, such as neuraxial anesthesia, maternal medication exposure, and meconium, may play a role in the interpretation of category II FHT. Future EFM studies should further target FHT patterns predictive of neonatal morbidity and explore the utility of intrauterine resuscitation techniques for specific subgroups.

REFERENCES

1. Chen HY, Chauhan SP, Ananth CV, et al. Electronic fetal heart rate monitoring and its relationship to neonatal and infant mortality in the United States. Am J Obstet Gynecol 2011;204(6):491.e1-10.

2. Boyle A, Reddy UM, Landy HJ, et al. Primary cesarean delivery in the United States. Obstet Gynecol 2013;122(1):33–40.

3. Ananth CV, Chauhan SP, Chen HY, et al. Electronic fetal monitoring in the United States: temporal trends and adverse perinatal outcomes. Obstet Gynecol 2013; 121(5):927–33.

4. Vintzileos AM, Nochimson DJ, Guzman ER, et al. Intrapartum electronic fetal heart rate monitoring versus intermittent auscultation: a meta-analysis. Obstet Gynecol 1995;85(1):149–55.

5. Vintzileos AM, Antsaklis A, Varvarigos I, et al. A randomized trial of intrapartum electronic fetal heart rate monitoring versus intermittent auscultation. Obstet Gynecol 1993;81(6):899–907.

6. Alfirevic Z, Devane D, Gyte GM. Continuous cardiotocography (CTG) as a form of electronic fetal monitoring (EFM) for fetal assessment during labour. Cochrane Database Syst Rev 2013;(5):CD006066.

7. Leveno KJ, Cunningham FG, Nelson S, et al. A prospective comparison of selective and universal electronic fetal monitoring in 34,995 pregnancies. N Engl J Med 1986;315(10):615–9.

8. Vintzileos AM, Nochimson DJ, Antsaklis A, et al. Comparison of intrapartum electronic fetal heart rate monitoring versus intermittent auscultation in detecting fetal acidemia at birth. Am J Obstet Gynecol 1995;173(4):1021–4.

9. Clark SL, Hamilton EF, Garite TJ, et al. The limits of electronic fetal heart rate monitoring in the prevention of neonatal metabolic acidemia. Am J Obstet Gynecol 2017;216(2):163.e1-6.

10. Macones GA, Hankins GD, Spong CY, et al. The 2008 National Institute of Child Health and Human Development workshop report on electronic fetal monitoring: update on definitions, interpretation, and research guidelines. Obstet Gynecol 2008;112(3):661–6.

11. American College of Obstetricians and Gynecologists. Practice bulletin no. 116: Management of intrapartum fetal heart rate tracings. Obstet Gynecol 2010; 116(5):1232–40.

12. Blackwell SC, Grobman WA, Antoniewicz L, et al. Interobserver and intraobserver reliability of the NICHD 3-Tier fetal heart rate interpretation system. Am J Obstet Gynecol 2011;205(4):378.e1-5.

13. Cahill AG, Roehl KA, Odibo AO, et al. Association and prediction of neonatal acidemia. Am J Obstet Gynecol 2012;207(3):206.e1-8.

14. Low JA, Victory R, Derrick EJ. Predictive value of electronic fetal monitoring for intrapartum fetal asphyxia with metabolic acidosis. Obstet Gynecol 1999;93(2): 285–91.

15. Williams KP, Galerneau F. Intrapartum fetal heart rate patterns in the prediction of neonatal acidemia. Am J Obstet Gynecol 2003;188(3):820–3.

16. Cahill AG, Spain J. Intrapartum fetal monitoring. Clin Obstet Gynecol 2015;58(2): 263–8.

17. Clark SL, Gimovsky ML, Miller FC. The scalp stimulation test: a clinical alternative to fetal scalp blood sampling. Am J Obstet Gynecol 1984;148(3):274–7.

18. Elimian A, Figueroa R, Tejani N. Intrapartum assessment of fetal well-being: a comparison of scalp stimulation with scalp blood pH sampling. Obstet Gynecol 1997;89(3):373–6.

19. Smith CV, Nguyen HN, Phelan JP, et al. Intrapartum assessment of fetal well-being: a comparison of fetal acoustic stimulation with acid-base determinations. Am J Obstet Gynecol 1986;155(4):726–8.

20. Chandraharan E. Fetal scalp blood sampling during labour: is it a useful diagnostic test or a historical test that no longer has a place in modern clinical obstetrics? BJOG 2014;121(9):1056–60 [discussion: 1060–2].

21. Sherman DJ, Arieli S, Raziel A, et al. The effect of sampling technique on measurement of fetal blood pH and gases–an in vitro system. Am J Obstet Gynecol 1994;171(4):1125–8.

22. Clark SL, Paul RH. Intrapartum fetal surveillance: the role of fetal scalp blood sampling. Am J Obstet Gynecol 1985;153(7):717–20.

23. Yam J, Chua S, Arulkumaran S. Intrapartum fetal pulse oximetry. Part I: Principles and technical issues. Obstet Gynecol Surv 2000;55(3):163–72.
24. Bloom SL, Spong CY, Thom E, et al. Fetal pulse oximetry and cesarean delivery. N Engl J Med 2006;355(21):2195–202.
25. East CE, Begg L, Colditz PB, et al. Fetal pulse oximetry for fetal assessment in labour. Cochrane Database Syst Rev 2014;(10):CD004075.
26. Belfort MA, Saade GR, Thom E, et al. A randomized trial of intrapartum fetal ECG ST-segment analysis. N Engl J Med 2015;373(7):632–41.
27. Neilson JP. Fetal electrocardiogram (ECG) for fetal monitoring during labour. Cochrane Database Syst Rev 2015;(12):CD000116.
28. Harper LM, Shanks AL, Tuuli MG, et al. The risks and benefits of internal monitors in laboring patients. Am J Obstet Gynecol 2013;209(1):38.e1-6.
29. Kawakita T, Reddy UM, Landy HJ, et al. Neonatal complications associated with use of fetal scalp electrode: a retrospective study. BJOG 2016;123(11): 1797–803.
30. Miyazaki FS, Nevarez F. Saline amnioinfusion for relief of repetitive variable decelerations: a prospective randomized study. Am J Obstet Gynecol 1985;153(3): 301–6.
31. Hofmeyr GJ, Lawrie TA. Amnioinfusion for potential or suspected umbilical cord compression in labour. Cochrane Database Syst Rev 2012;1:CD000013.
32. Pitt C, Sanchez-Ramos L, Kaunitz AM, et al. Prophylactic amnioinfusion for intrapartum oligohydramnios: a meta-analysis of randomized controlled trials. Obstet Gynecol 2000;96(5 Pt 2):861–6.
33. Strong TH Jr, Hetzler G, Sarno AP, et al. Prophylactic intrapartum amnioinfusion: a randomized clinical trial. Am J Obstet Gynecol 1990;162(6):1370–4 [discussion: 1374–5].
34. Owen J, Henson BV, Hauth JC. A prospective randomized study of saline solution amnioinfusion. Am J Obstet Gynecol 1990;162(5):1146–9.
35. Carbonne B, Benachi A, Leveque ML, et al. Maternal position during labor: effects on fetal oxygen saturation measured by pulse oximetry. Obstet Gynecol 1996;88(5):797–800.
36. Heuser CC, Knight S, Esplin MS, et al. Tachysystole in term labor: incidence, risk factors, outcomes, and effect on fetal heart tracings. Am J Obstet Gynecol 2013; 209(1):32.e1-6.
37. Stewart RD, Bleich AT, Lo JY, et al. Defining uterine tachysystole: how much is too much? Am J Obstet Gynecol 2012;207(4):290.e1-6.
38. Althabe O Jr, Schwarcz RL, Pose SV, et al. Effects on fetal heart rate and fetal pO_2 of oxygen administration to the mother. Am J Obstet Gynecol 1967;98(6): 858–70.
39. Young DC, Popat R, Luther ER, et al. Influence of maternal oxygen administration on the term fetus before labor. Am J Obstet Gynecol 1980;136(3):321–4.
40. Khaw KS, Wang CC, Ngan Kee WD, et al. Effects of high inspired oxygen fraction during elective caesarean section under spinal anaesthesia on maternal and fetal oxygenation and lipid peroxidation. Br J Anaesth 2002;88(1):18–23.
41. Ramanathan S, Gandhi S, Arismendy J, et al. Oxygen transfer from mother to fetus during cesarean section under epidural anesthesia. Anesth Analg 1982; 61(7):576–81.
42. Raghuraman N, Temming LA, Stout MJ, et al. Intrauterine hyperoxemia and risk of neonatal morbidity. Obstet Gynecol 2017;129(4):676–82.
43. Hamel MS, Anderson BL, Rouse DJ. Oxygen for intrauterine resuscitation: of unproved benefit and potentially harmful. Am J Obstet Gynecol 2014;211(2):124–7.

44. American College of Obstetricians and Gynecologists. ACOG Practice Bulletin No. 106: Intrapartum fetal heart rate monitoring: nomenclature, interpretation, and general management principles. Obstet Gynecol 2009;114(1):192–202.

45. Simmons SW, Cyna AM, Dennis AT, et al. Combined spinal-epidural versus epidural analgesia in labour. Cochrane Database Syst Rev 2007;(3):CD003401.

46. Patel NP, El-Wahab N, Fernando R, et al. Fetal effects of combined spinal-epidural vs epidural labour analgesia: a prospective, randomised double-blind study. Anaesthesia 2014;69(5):458–67.

47. Abrao KC, Francisco RP, Miyadahira S, et al. Elevation of uterine basal tone and fetal heart rate abnormalities after labor analgesia: a randomized controlled trial. Obstet Gynecol 2009;113(1):41–7.

48. Steiger RM, Nageotte MP. Effect of uterine contractility and maternal hypotension on prolonged decelerations after bupivacaine epidural anesthesia. Am J Obstet Gynecol 1990;163(3):808–12.

49. Hattler J, Klimek M, Rossaint R, et al. The effect of combined spinal-epidural versus epidural analgesia in laboring women on nonreassuring fetal heart rate tracings: systematic review and meta-analysis. Anesth Analg 2016;123(4): 955–64.

50. Kahn L, Hubert E. Combined spinal epidural (CSE) analgesia, fetal bradycardia, and uterine hypertonus. Reg Anesth pain Med 1998;23(1):111–2.

51. Palmer CM, Maciulla JE, Cork RC, et al. The incidence of fetal heart rate changes after intrathecal fentanyl labor analgesia. Anesth Analg 1999;88(3):577–81.

52. Stewart AM, Macones GA, Odibo AO, et al. Changes in fetal heart tracing characteristics after magnesium exposure. Am J Perinatol 2014;31(10):869–74.

53. Wright JW, Ridgway LE, Wright BD, et al. Effect of MgSO4 on heart rate monitoring in the preterm fetus. J Reprod Med 1996;41(8):605–8.

54. Sameshima H, Ikenoue T, Kamitomo M, et al. Effects of 4 hours magnesium sulfate infusion on fetal heart rate variability and reactivity in a goat model. Am J Perinatol 1998;15(9):535–8.

55. Hallak M, Martinez-Poyer J, Kruger ML, et al. The effect of magnesium sulfate on fetal heart rate parameters: A randomized, placebo-controlled trial. Am J Obstet Gynecol 1999;181(5 Pt 1):1122–7.

56. Twickler DM, McIntire DD, Alexander JM, et al. Effects of magnesium sulfate on preterm fetal cerebral blood flow using Doppler analysis: a randomized controlled trial. Obstet Gynecol 2010;115(1):21–5.

57. Gagnon R, Hunse C, Bocking AD. Fetal heart rate patterns in the small-for-gestational-age human fetus. Am J Obstet Gynecol 1989;161(3):779–84.

58. Vinkesteijn AS, Struijk PC, Ursem NT, et al. Fetal heart rate and umbilical artery flow velocity variability in intrauterine growth restriction: a matched controlled study. Ultrasound Obstet Gynecol 2004;23(5):461–5.

59. Epplin KA, Tuuli MG, Odibo AO, et al. Effect of growth restriction on fetal heart rate patterns in the second stage of labor. Am J Perinatol 2015;32(9):873–8.

60. Frey HA, Tuuli MG, Shanks AL, et al. Interpreting category II fetal heart rate tracings: does meconium matter? Am J Obstet Gynecol 2014;211(6):644.e1-8.

61. Xu H, Mas-Calvet M, Wei SQ, et al. Abnormal fetal heart rate tracing patterns in patients with thick meconium staining of the amniotic fluid: association with perinatal outcomes. Am J Obstet Gynecol 2009;200(3):283.e1-7.

62. Das AK, Jana N, Dasgupta S, et al. Intrapartum transcervical amnioinfusion for meconium-stained amniotic fluid. Int J Gynaecol Obstet 2007;97(3):182–6.

63. Fraser WD, Hofmeyr J, Lede R, et al. Amnioinfusion for the prevention of the meconium aspiration syndrome. N Engl J Med 2005;353(9):909–17.

The Evolution of the Laborist

Allison J. Allen, MD*, Aaron B. Caughey, MD, PhD

KEYWORDS

• Laborist • Obstetric hospitalist • Labor outcomes • Economic impact

KEY POINTS

- The laborist movement, although relatively new, is rapidly expanding as a means to improve patient care and physician burnout and decrease malpractice claims.
- Although there are many different models of laborists, full-time laborists may have a greater impact on improvement in obstetric outcomes.
- Full-time laborists are found to decrease rates of cesarean delivery; however, their impact on other maternal or neonatal morbidity markers is unknown.
- The use of laborists can decrease rates of malpractice claims and litigation, not only through the immediate availability of physicians for emergent scenarios but through improved care in uncertain clinical scenarios.

INTRODUCTION

Historically, a patient's physician in the outpatient setting would follow up with the patient and provide care in the inpatient setting as well. However, throughout the latter quarter of the 20th century, hospitalizations became increasingly complicated with multiple tests and treatments needing to be ordered, interpreted, and responded to in rapid succession. Similarly, patients in the outpatient environment have also increased in complexity, and the demands on physicians balancing both the outpatient and inpatient medicine became more challenging. The hospitalist movement was formally introduced in 1996 by Robert Watcher.[1] The hospitalist was introduced as a way to improve the quality of care patients receive, to decrease hospital costs by shortening length of stay, and to improve physician quality of life.

In obstetrics, the concept of the laborist was first described by Weinstein[2] in 2003 as an offshoot to the hospitalist movement, although this kind of coverage had been used in large Health Maintenance Organization practices such as Kaiser Permanente since

Disclosure Statement: The authors have no commercial or financial disclosures or conflicts of interest.
Department of Obstetrics and Gynecology, Oregon Health & Science University, 3181 SW Sam Jackson Park Road, L466, Portland, OR 97239-3098, USA
* Corresponding author.
E-mail address: landstro@ohsu.edu

Obstet Gynecol Clin N Am 44 (2017) 625–629
http://dx.doi.org/10.1016/j.ogc.2017.08.001
0889-8545/17/© 2017 Elsevier Inc. All rights reserved.

obgyn.theclinics.com

the 1990s. This concept represented a dramatic shift in the way in which obstetric care was provided. Previously, obstetricians had to simultaneously balance a full office practice with the demands of patients admitted to the labor suite. Additionally, many obstetricians took frequent night call, with solo practice clinicians being on call every night except on the rare vacation. The laborist provided a model to hand off the demands of the labor suite to physicians whose sole responsibility was the care of women in labor, while improving care and decreasing rates of physician burnout.[2]

Since the introduction of the laborist more than 10 years ago, this specialty role has gained momentum and traction, particularly in large hospitals with high-volume labor and delivery suites. In a 2010 statement, the American College of Obstetricians and Gynecologists (ACOG) released a statement supporting "the continued development of the obstetric-gynecologic hospitalist model as one potential approach to achieving increased professional and patient satisfaction while maintaining safe and effective care across delivery settings".[3] Later that same year, 25% of ACOG member responders identified themselves as either a laborist or hospitalist.[4] In another 2010 study surveying National Perinatal Information Center/Quality Analytic Services member hospitals, approximately 40% were employing laborists.[5] By 2011, the Society of OB/Gyn Hospitalists formed and by 2016 had 600 dues-paying members. In part, the evolution of the laborist movement was founded on improving provider job satisfaction and decreasing rates of physician burnout. In the same 2010 survey of ACOG members, those who self-identified as laborists or hospitalists were asked to rate their job satisfaction. More than 92% rated themselves between satisfied and extremely satisfied.[4]

Although the laborist movement has expanded, there does not exist a standardized definition of what laborist coverage looks like. Similarly, there are minimal data on maternal and neonatal outcomes or differences in rates of litigation. This article reviews models of laborist care, discusses the potential benefits in quality of maternal care, and discusses the potential financial impact of this care model.

MODELS OF CARE

In the original model presented by Weinstein,[2] the labor suite would be covered by 4 physicians working no more than 14 hours in a shift. This was, he argued, to minimize fatigue and optimize the care provided to patients. Since this original recommendation, the role of the laborist and the physician who fulfills that role has varied greatly between hospitals.

In the traditional model, a group of laborists are hired by the hospital to cover the labor and delivery unit within the hospital. Commonly, the laborist groups care for patients belonging to certain private groups along with patients without a designated provider such as those admitted to a hospital that is different from where they received prenatal care. These physicians are also readily available to manage obstetric emergencies or precipitous deliveries of patients belonging to other practices. Additionally, this role can be expanded to cover the hospital's gynecologic emergencies and consultations. In a variation of this model, some laborist groups primarily cover the labor suite and gynecologic consults in the emergency department with a small proportion of their time being spent in an outpatient clinic.

Another model shares shift work within large practice groups or between multiple small practice groups, also called *community laborists*. In this model, private practice physicians occasionally cover labor and delivery for 12- or 24-hour shifts. During their laborist shift, they don't have clinical responsibilities and thus can provide complete coverage of both routine and emergency situations for all participating groups. One downside to this model of care is the sporadic nature to which these physicians are working in the labor suite, which does not increase the expertise or the comfort level of the provider within this role.

QUALITY OF CARE

As the role of laborists expanded and permeated into the everyday care of women in labor and delivery, questions arose about the quality of care being provided. Specific concerns regarded increasing patient hand-offs, difficulty with transition of care from a patient's primary outpatient obstetrician/gynecologist to an inpatient specialist, and unknown effects of the transition on maternal and neonatal morbidity and mortality.[6] However, an increasing body of evidence suggests that, similar to improved care outcomes in the hospitalist literature, patient care improves with use of laborists.

One study retrospectively looked at more than 6000 term, nulliparous deliveries in one hospital during 3 different coverage types: traditional, community laborists, and full-time laborists. They showed 27% and 23% reduction in cesarean delivery rates with full-time laborists when compared with the periods with traditional and community laborist coverage, respectively.[7] Additionally, a study at a single hospital that examined outcomes after the adoption of a laborist program found that women who were cared for under the traditional model had an 86% higher chance of a cesarean delivery.[8] There are varying hypotheses regarding the specific attributes of a laborist model that account for such dramatic differences in the cesarean delivery rate, which has been largely stagnant over the last 10 years, and there are likely several factors at play.

In traditional models, physicians are constantly balancing their time between clinical duties, such as office and surgical responsibilities, and the actively laboring patient. Given these demands on their time, it is likely that physicians change their practice decisions and habits to accommodate their clinical responsibilities. Additionally, the differences seen between rates of cesarean delivery among laborists and community laborists within the same hospital suggest that the type of laborist matters.[7] Community laborists take laborist calls infrequently; thus, although they are available more readily for obstetric emergencies, their practice pattern is likely not dramatically different from that of private physicians. Finally, one cannot discount the experiential difference of practitioners whose sole responsibility is the management of labor and delivery and their increased comfort and patience with fetal heart rate tracings of unknown significance and clinical uncertainty.

Patient satisfaction with the care they receive from laborists has also been questioned, with providers concerned that patients will be unhappy to have their delivery performed by a physician they have never met. However, although this may be true in certain practice settings, in one survey of patients before and after the implementation of a laborist care model, there was no difference in patient satisfaction.[9]

There continues to be minimal information on neonatal outcome differences with the use of a laborist model. This lack of data is likely caused by low prevalence of term neonatal morbidity/mortality and difficulty discerning true causation. However, one could postulate that with 24-hour coverage of labor and delivery, there would be increased responsiveness to obstetric emergencies such as abruption, cord prolapse, and uterine rupture.

FINANCIAL IMPACT

The implementation of a laborist model can be costly upfront for health systems to enact, with one group estimating 1.25 to 1.5 million dollars for the employment of

4.5 full-time laborists.[10] There are many models of cost-distribution, with health care systems (eg, Kaiser Permanente), hospitals, or subspecialty groups (eg, maternal-fetal medicine) either fully funding or sharing the costs. Similarly, the way in which laborists bill for their time has also been a point of discussion. In the National Perinatal Information Center/Quality Analytic Services survey of hospitalists, 56% were hired as salaried employees, 32% performed traditional physician billing, and 24% performed hospital-based billing.[5]

One potential economic benefit offsetting these costs are the potential for subsequent decreased malpractice claims and litigation. The wide practice variation seen in traditional private practice coverage of labor and delivery leads to a decrease in the quality of care patients receive and potential for increased litigation. For example, a study of a large hospital system in 2008 showed that 70% of obstetric malpractice claims involved substandard care and were ultimately responsible for 79% of the costs associated with those claims. They subsequently concluded that a significant proportion of these could have been avoided with continuous in-house labor coverage.[11] Similarly, in a review of almost 200 closed malpractice claims, 40% were related to intrapartum fetal hypoxia, many of which might have been avoidable with immediately available intervention.[12]

Another way in which the laborist model can contribute to lowering health care costs overall is through increasing availability of trial of labor after cesarean (TOLAC). TOLAC is found to be cost effective when compared with repeat cesarean delivery, with a cost savings of $164 million per 100,000 women.[13] However, many hospitals are unable to offer TOLAC, even to women who are excellent candidates, because of the 1999 ACOG recommendation for physicians to be "immediately available" during TOLAC.[14] Implementation of a laborist model provides this safety checkpoint for the hospital, as well as mitigating malpractice concerns.

SUMMARY

The laborist model of care has been rapidly expanding since its introduction in 2003. This care model, although still in its relative infancy, has thus far been found to potentially decrease rates of cesarean delivery, improve physician job satisfaction, and decrease medical malpractice claims. Overall, there have been relatively few studies on the laborist model of care, particularly as it relates to maternal and neonatal morbidity and mortality. As this model of care continues to expand and develop, more work on its optimization and potential benefits needs to be done.

REFERENCES

1. Watcher RM, Goldman L. The emerging role of "hospitalists" in the American health care system. N Engl J Med 1996;335(7):514–7.
2. Weinstein L. The laborist: a new focus of practice for the obstetrician. Am J Obstet Gynecol 2003;188:310–2.
3. American College of Obstetricians and Gynecologists. Committee opinion no. 459: the obstetric-gynecologic hospitalist. Obstet Gynecol 2010;116:237–9.
4. Funk C, Anderson BL, Schulkin J, et al. Survey of obstetric and gynecologic hospitalists and laborists. Am J Obstet Gynecol 2010;203(2):177.
5. Srinivas SK, Shocksnider J, Caldwell D, et al. Laborist model of care: who is using it? J Matern Fetal Neonatal Med 2012;25(3):257–60.
6. Srinivas SK, Lorch SA. The laborist model of obstetric care: we need more evidence. Am J Obstet Gynecol 2012;7:30–5.

7. Iriye BK, Huang WH, Condon J, et al. Implementation of a laborist program and evaluation of the effect upon cesarean delivery. Am J Obstet Gynecol 2013; 209(3):251.

8. Nijagal MA, Kupperman M, Nakagawa S, et al. Two practice models in one labor and delivery unit: association with cesarean delivery rates. Am J Obstet Gynecol 2015;212(4):491.

9. Srinivas SK, Jesus AO, Turbo A, et al. Patient satisfaction with the laborist model of care in a large urban hospital. Patient Prefer Adherence 2013;7:217–22.

10. Olson R, Garite TJ, Fishman A, et al. Obstetrician/gynecologist hospitalists: can we improved safety and outcomes for patients and hospitals and improve lifestyle for physicians? Am J Obstet Gynecol 2012;207(2):81–6.

11. Clark SL, Belfort MA, Dildy GA, et al. Reducing obstetric litigation through alterations in practice patterns. Obstet Gynecol 2008;112:1279–83.

12. Clark SL, Belfort MA, Dildy GA. Reducing obstetric litigation through alterations in practice patterns - experience with 189 closed claims. Am J Obstet Gynecol 2006;195:s118.

13. Gilbert SA, Grobman WA, Landon MB, et al. Lifetime cost-effectiveness of trial of labor after cesarean in the United States. Value Health 2013;16(6):953–64.

14. American College of Obstetricians and Gynecologists. Vaginal delivery after previous cesarean section. Washington, DC: ACOG; 1999. Practice Bulletin Number 5.

Fetal Malpresentation and Malposition

Diagnosis and Management

Rachel A. Pilliod, MD*, Aaron B. Caughey, MD, PhD

KEYWORDS

- Fetal malposition • Fetal malpresentation • Occiput posterior • Manual rotation
- Assisted vaginal delivery

KEY POINTS

- Fetal malpresentation includes breech, shoulder, compound, face, and brow presentations.
- Risk factors for fetal malposition include multiple fetal and maternal factors, including fetal size, amniotic fluid volume, fetal anomalies, maternal habitus, and pelvic structure.
- Breech presentation is the most commonly encountered fetal malpresentation and may be managed with external cephalic version or planned cesarean delivery. Planned vaginal delivery for breech presentation is associated with adverse perinatal outcomes and is therefore only considered in selective cases with experienced providers and well-informed patients.
- Fetal malposition includes occiput posterior and occiput transverse, is a commonly occurring problem in obstetrics, and can be diagnosed in active labor by clinical examination or bedside ultrasound.
- Most occiput posterior and occiput transverse cases will spontaneously rotate to occiput anterior at the time of delivery; however, persistent occiput posterior and occiput transverse may be managed with manual or digital rotation, which has high success rates and minimal adverse effects.

INTRODUCTION

Spontaneous vaginal delivery is most common when a cephalic-presenting (head down) fetus is in the occiput anterior position. When the fetal head is occiput anterior and flexed, the fetal head diameter is minimized and the presenting shape optimized to fit through the pelvis. Most fetuses at term present head down and flexed with the fetal occiput anterior. When the fetus deviates from this presentation or position, it can

Department of Obstetrics and Gynecology, Oregon Health & Science University, 3181 Southwest Sam Jackson Park Road, Portland, OR 97239, USA
* Corresponding author. 3181 Southwest Sam Jackson Park Road, Mail Code L466, Portland, OR 97239.
E-mail address: pilliodr@ohsu.edu

Obstet Gynecol Clin N Am 44 (2017) 631–643
http://dx.doi.org/10.1016/j.ogc.2017.08.003
0889-8545/17/© 2017 Elsevier Inc. All rights reserved.

obgyn.theclinics.com

provide a challenging clinical situation for even experienced providers. When a fetus is in a noncephalic or nonvertex presentation, it is considered malpresentation. Fetal malposition is a term used to describe a fetus that is rotated so that it is in the occiput posterior or occiput transverse positions. Both of these conditions are associated with increased rates of adverse maternal and perinatal events, including cesarean delivery. In a time when reduction of primary cesarean deliveries remains a priority for providers, health care systems, and patients, identifying these conditions along with the opportunities and pitfalls associated with diagnosis and management is an area of active discussion in clinical practice.[1,2]

FETAL MALPRESENTATION

Fetal presentation refers to the fetal anatomic part proceeding first into and through the pelvic inlet. Most commonly, the fetal head is presenting, which is referred to as cephalic presentation. Once cervical dilation has occurred and the fetal fontanels may be appreciated, if the head is flexed, the presenting anatomy of the fetal head is just in front of the posterior fontanel, also known as the fetal vertex. The fetal vertex is really an area, not just a point, and is bounded anteriorly by the anterior fontanel and posteriorly by the posterior fontanel. Most commonly, women in active labor will have a fetus in the vertex presentation. Any circumstance where the fetal presenting part is other than the vertex is considered malpresentation, including breech presentation, transverse and oblique lie with shoulder presentation, face and brow presentation, and compound (hand or arm) presentation. The prevalence, complications, diagnosis, and management of each are reviewed.

Breech Presentation

Breech presentation refers to a fetus with the feet or buttocks presenting in the pelvic inlet and is the most common type of malpresentation.[3,4] It is further categorized by the presenting fetal part in relationship to the maternal pelvis:

- Frank breech: the fetus is in a pike position with the buttocks presenting and the hips flexed, but knees extended.
- Complete breech: the fetus has both knees and hips flexed so the feet are near the buttocks, but the buttocks are presenting.
- Incomplete breech: the fetus has either one or both knees flexed and one or both hips flexed resulting in either the feet or the knee below the buttock.
- Footling breech: a type of incomplete breech wherein the fetus has one or both feet presenting.

Diagnosis is made if breech presentation is suspected on Leopold examination or digital examination if the cervix is dilated and may be confirmed by ultrasound. Breech presentation affects approximately 3% to 4% of deliveries with the incidence decreasing with advancing gestational age.[4–6] In addition to prematurity, fetal factors associated with breech presentation include aneuploidy and congenital anomalies, growth restriction, multiple gestation, and female fetal sex.[7–9] Maternal characteristics include uterine anomalies, uterine fibroids, prior cesarean delivery, older maternal age, multiparity, prior pregnancy with breech presentation, and placenta previa.[6,10,11]

Significant outcomes associated with breech presentation under current practice in the developed world are largely associated with mode of delivery as well as the underlying fetal and maternal conditions predisposing to breech presentation. However, it should be noted that there is an independent association with breech presentation and stillbirth compared with cephalic-presenting fetuses.[12,13] Risks associated with laboring or rupture of membranes in a breech presentation are significant and portend adverse outcomes for the fetus, including severe morbidity and mortality. The risk of adverse obstetric outcomes with breech presentation includes cord prolapse and prolonged cord compression in the setting of rupture of membranes. If the fetus delivers vaginally with the breech presentation, there is a risk for head entrapment as well as for birth trauma associated with maneuvers for delivery of the later coming head.[14,15]

Given these risks, vaginal breech delivery in singleton pregnancies is not routinely advised in the United States. In light of efforts to reduce primary cesarean deliveries, and with attention paid to subsequent pregnancies, external cephalic version (ECV) may be attempted in women with a breech-presenting fetus. ECV is a procedure in which a breech-presenting fetus is manually rotated to cephalic presentation by applying pressure and direction through the maternal gravid abdomen. ECV is successful in approximately 50% to 65% of cases, and offering this for women without contraindications with breech-presenting fetus is recommended.[16-18] Favorable characteristics include multiparity, normal amniotic fluid volume, unengaged presenting fetal part, earlier gestation (34–36 weeks), regional anesthesia, and multiparity.[16-20] Use of uterine tocolysis and regional anesthesia have also been associated with successful ECV.[17,19,20] Factors associated with unsuccessful ECV include nulliparity, low amniotic fluid volume, maternal obesity, advanced gestation, excessive estimated fetal weight, posterior located fetal spine and anterior or lateral placenta, and ECV attempt at term.[16-20] In counseling patients, risks of the procedure including placental abruption, cord prolapse, rupture of membranes, and emergency cesarean delivery should be reviewed, although the overall risk of complications is estimated to be approximately 6%.[21]

Delivery planning for women with fetuses in the breech presentation primarily focuses on improving perinatal morbidity and mortality. Current practice is guided by the Term Breech Trial, published in 2000, which is an international randomized controlled trial. The Term Breech Trial randomly assigned complete and frank presenting fetuses to planned vaginal or planned cesarean delivery. Perinatal mortality, neonatal mortality, and serious neonatal morbidity were lower in women with a planned cesarean delivery (relative risk 0.33, 95% confidence interval 0.19–0.59; $P<.0001$).[22] Since that time, vaginal breech deliveries have continued to decrease. Follow-up studies have been published and suggest that outcomes at 2 years after birth were not different for women or infants born to either arm of the trial.[23,24] It has been suggested that the absence of difference at 2 years is due to the study being underpowered to appreciate the differences. Alternatively, it may be that the short-term outcomes examined in the original study with the composite morbidity and mortality outcome overestimated the risk associated with vaginal breech delivery.

Subsequent studies have suggested that attempted planned vaginal breech deliveries with select patients may not negatively impact neonatal outcomes.[25-27] Suggested criteria for trial of vaginal breech delivery include singleton, nonanomalous pregnancies with frank or complete breech at term with an estimated fetal weight of 2500 to 4000 g, and a flexed fetal head. In addition, clinical examination with or without imaging to assess the adequacy of the maternal pelvis is recommended.[27,28] Close monitoring of labor progression is necessary, and the provider experience and comfort with vaginal breech deliveries should not be underestimated. Also, women should be appropriately counseled about the risks and benefits of the procedure relative to a planned cesarean delivery.

Transverse and Oblique Lie

Oblique and transverse lie most often result in the fetal shoulder as the deepest presenting part and affects approximately 0.03% of deliveries.[29] Diagnosis is made by Leopold maneuver and by ultrasound examination. These presentations are most often seen in conditions whereby the fetus is small, from growth restriction or prematurity, or the uterus is compliant as in the case of high parity. As such, adverse outcomes are associated with oblique and transverse presentation, although the underlying prematurity and low birth weight may serve confounding factors in some cases.[30] Cord prolapse is also associated with these presentations, which is associated with adverse outcomes as described with breech presentation.[31] ECV may be attempted if the condition is diagnosed before rupture of membranes or labor, but cesarean delivery is indicated if active labor or rupture of membranes is present.

Face and Brow Presentation

Face and brow presentations occur when the fetus is cephalic presenting, but the fetal neck is extended so that the vertex is not presenting. Both face and brow presentations are relatively uncommon with an incidence of 0.1% to 0.2% of all deliveries and are associated with nulliparity, cephalopelvic disproportion, black race/ethnicity, prematurity, fetal growth disorders (both low birth weight and fetal macrosomia), and fetal anomalies.[32–34] Both are associated with fetal soft tissue trauma, including bruising and edema at the presenting part as well as increased rates of cesarean delivery.[35] Diagnosis is made by digital examination in labor with palpation of facial parts. The chin is not palpable in brow presentation, but it is with a face presentation and is used to further characterize the fetal position that is described as mentum (chin) anterior, mentum transverse, or mentum posterior. In the case of mentum posterior face presentation, vaginal delivery requires neck extension beyond what is physiologically possible for the fetus. Should spontaneous rotation or flexion not occur, manual assistance is not recommended because of considerable risks, including uterine rupture, cord prolapse, and spinal trauma to the fetus.[34,36] Brow, mentum anterior, and mentum transverse presentations may be monitored in labor, and most will deliver spontaneously; however, early consideration of cesarean delivery for prolonged or abnormal labor is indicated.[34,37]

Compound Presentation

A fetus presenting with an extremity preceding or adjacent to the fetal head is described as compound presentation. Most often being a hand or arm, a compound presentation affects approximately 0.1% to 0.2% of deliveries.[38,39] Diagnosis is made on digital vaginal examination with palpation of the involved extremity. Compound presentation is associated with prematurity and low birth weight, high amniotic fluid levels (polyhydramnios), and multiple gestation.[38,39] Not surprisingly, cord prolapse is also increased in cases of compound presentation. Although uncommon, limb trauma of the presenting fetal part and maternal trauma, including rectal injury, have been described, mostly as case reports in the available, recent literature.[40–42] Identification of compound presentation early in labor may be managed expectantly because the fetal part may be retracted as the fetal head engages the pelvis and spontaneous delivery may occur. In cases of persistent compound presentation with prolonged labor, gentle reduction with upward pressure of the presenting fetal part may be attempted. In cases of labor dystocia, whereby the fetal limb cannot be moved or concern for injury to the presenting fetal part, cesarean delivery is indicated.

FETAL MALPOSITION

Occiput posterior position is defined as the fetal occiput being oriented to the posterior maternal pelvis. Occiput transverse position is defined as the fetal sagittal suture and fontanels aligned in the transverse maternal pelvis. The fetal position can be further specified relative to the maternal pelvis, including the right and left side with left occiput transverse and right occiput transverse, and right occiput posterior and left occiput posterior for when the occiput is posterior but deviates from the midline up to 45° in either direction. Persistent occiput posterior is when the malposition is maintained during the second stage until delivery. Although occiput posterior and occiput transverse positions may be observed in early and active labor, the persistence of these positions in the second stage through delivery are associated with adverse outcomes, including cesarean delivery.

Prevalence

Persistent occiput posterior has been estimated to affect between 1.8% and 12.9% of pregnancies and occiput transverse at delivery varied from 0.2% to 8.1% of pregnancies.[43–48] In the first stage of labor, left occiput posterior is observed more frequently than right occiput posterior, which are both more prevalent than direct occiput posterior.[49] In the second stage of labor, right occiput posterior is noted most frequently followed by left occiput posterior and then direct occiput posterior.[50] At what point in labor the malposition is identified is of significance because most occiput posterior and occiput transverse identified in early labor and at the onset of the second stage rotate to occiput anterior without intervention. Persistent malposition at birth has been associated with nulliparity, African American race, maternal age greater than 35 years, short maternal stature, induction of labor and oxytocin augmentation, anterior placenta, advancing gestational age (41 weeks and beyond), and fetal macrosomia (>4000 g).[43,45,51,52] The presence of a narrow suprapubic arch on ultrasound evaluation has been associated with persistent occiput posterior at birth in one small study.[52] In addition, women with a prior pregnancy affected by occiput posterior position at birth have an increased risk for persistent occiput posterior in subsequent pregnancies compared with women with prior birth in the occiput anterior position, suggesting the maternal bony pelvis plays a considerable, nonmodifiable role in fetal position.[53]

The role of epidural anesthesia and the persistence of occiput posterior remain points of discussion. Multiple retrospective studies have suggested an association between persistent occiput posterior and epidural use with authors and clinicians theorizing a causal role mediated by pelvic floor relaxation in the presence of epidural anesthesia.[43,45] One prospective study examined changes in fetal position during labor in nulliparous women using serial ultrasound examinations and observed the proportion of fetal occiput posterior position was equivalent at time of epidural placement and in early active labor (4 hours after admission) in women who did not have epidural analgesia; however, women who had epidural analgesia had a higher proportion of occiput posterior malposition at delivery (12.9%) compared with those without epidural (3.3%).[46] These observations led to the theory that epidural analgesia promotes pelvic muscle relaxation and thus inhibits fetal head rotation in labor, contributing to persistent occiput posterior position. However, a meta-analysis of the available randomized clinical trials did not show a statistically significant association, although available data were limited to 4 small trials.[54] Taking the meta-analysis into consideration, coupled with the observation that multiparous women with and without epidural anesthesia have a relaxed and accommodating pelvic floor and yet have considerably lower rates of persistent occiput posterior than nulliparous women, others have suggested that this causal theory is not well supported.[2]

Maternal and Neonatal Outcomes

Although overall prevalence of occiput posterior in labor is low, the impact on women and neonates is considerable. Compared with neonates delivering in the occiput anterior position, those in occiput posterior have higher rates of multiple adverse short-term outcomes, including 5-min Apgar scores less than 7, umbilical cord gas acidemia, neonatal intensive care unit admissions, and longer hospitalizations.[43] In addition, multiple studies have shown increased rates of birth trauma.[43,55] Interestingly, although it has been described that neonates delivering in the occiput posterior position have a lower rate of shoulder dystocia, they have a higher rate of brachial plexus injuries, which speaks to a cause related to malposition in labor as opposed to birth trauma at the time of delivery.[56]

It has been theorized that multiple factors contribute to these adverse outcomes, including longer labor, and with it higher incidence of chorioamnionitis. The increased rate of birth trauma is thought secondary to increased rates of operative deliveries or from the delivery itself based on the theory that occiput posterior is a manifestation of cephalopelvic disproportion. It is important to note that not all observational studies have been in agreement on the adverse outcomes observed in the short term for neonates, although study design and power differed.[43,44,51,55]

In terms of maternal complications, morbidity is often associated with duration of labor and mode of delivery. The persistence of occiput posterior to time of delivery has been associated with longer first and second stages of labor and the need for augmentation of labor.[44,51,55,57] Not surprisingly, the strength of the association of prolonged labor, particularly in the second stage, is greatest when occiput posterior is noticed in the second stage and persists.[2,55,58] Rates of operative delivery, both cesarean and operative vaginal delivery, are higher in women with persistent occiput posterior and occiput transverse on entry to the second stage of labor with highest rates among nulliparous women compared with their multiparous counterparts.[44,45,51,55] As expected with higher rates of labor dystocia, prolonged labor, and operative delivery rates, persistent occiput posterior is also associated with higher rates of postpartum hemorrhage or excessive blood loss.[51,59] In addition, cesarean delivery at the time of prolonged labor (>4 hours), delivery at full dilation, and cesarean in the setting of occiput posterior is associated with unintentional hysterotomy extension, which has associated increased operative time and morbidity.[59,60] Among women with vaginal delivery, perineal trauma is greater among occiput posterior and occiput transverse deliveries with higher rates of third- and fourth-degree lacerations.[51,55] Women with occiput posterior also face increased risk of infection with increased rates of chorioamnionitis and wound infection, although similar rates of endometritis.[51]

Diagnosis

Given the considerable perinatal morbidity associated with fetal malpresentation, accurate diagnosis is of considerable importance; however, timing of diagnosis is also important. Identification of fetal malposition in labor can occur at any point during the first and second stage of labor. Although most occiput posterior positions will rotate spontaneously to occiput anterior, the vast majority of occiput posterior at delivery is a consequence of unresolved occiput posterior rather than rotation from occiput anterior.[58,61] Diagnosis historically has been made clinically with a digital vaginal examination to assess the fetal sutures and fontanels relative to the maternal pelvis. Unfortunately, early vaginal digital assessment before full cervical dilation has been shown to be inaccurate up to 76% of the time when compared with ultrasound assessment, although this improved with increasing cervical dilation and advancing station.[49,62,63] In active labor, digital assessment proves more accurate; however, when compared with ultrasound, accuracy remains an issue with reports of 20% to 65% of clinical examinations revealing results inconsistent with concurrent ultrasound.[9,50,64–66] This inaccuracy is minimized by providing a greater degree of margin of error (±45°) and provider experience.

Intrapartum ultrasound relies upon correct identification of the fetal occiput by identifying the falx, orbits, or cerebellum and posterior fossa. This technique is most often taught as a transabdominal approach with the probe in the transverse alignment just superior to pubic symphysis. When the head is deeply engaged in the pelvis, transperineal or transvaginal approach may be used, but the landmarks for determining fetal position are the same. With such considerable superiority of ultrasound in intrapartum assessment of fetal position, if time permits, assessment with ultrasound to confirm position should be used before active management of labor and as a teaching aid for trainees in obstetrics.

Management

The first step in the management of occiput posterior and occiput transverse position is diagnosis and timing of diagnosis. Although identification of the fetal position should generally be performed in the active phase of the first stage, there are not generally interventions that have demonstrated benefit because most commonly the fetus will rotate to occiput anterior on its own. Multiple efforts have been made to identify maternal positions to reduce the rate of occiput posterior at time of delivery; the most extensively studied is a maternal hands and knees position with or without pelvic rocking. Although this has been proven successful in reducing maternal discomfort in the first stage of labor, it has not resulted in a reduction of persistent occiput posterior at the time of second stage or delivery.[67–70] More recently, lateral decubitus and hip abduction both individually and in combination with hands and knees have been trialed without significant impact on fetal position.[71,72]

If occiput posterior or occiput transverse is suspected at full dilation, close surveillance is initiated with efforts made to confirm position with ultrasound if available and to monitor progress in the second stage. Delayed pushing has been evaluated in small studies, but has not proven beneficial in minimizing occiput posterior at time of delivery.[55] Considering that even in the second stage most occiput posterior and occiput transverse presenting fetuses will spontaneously rotate,[73] if fetal heart tracing is reassuring, the authors' practice is to continue close monitoring for approximately 60 minutes for nulliparous women and 30 minutes for multiparous women before reevaluating progress. If delivery is not imminent, occiput posterior or occiput transverse is still suspected, and confirmation with bedside ultrasound has not occurred, then the authors recommend proceeding with ultrasound. At this point, they discuss with the patient a trial of manual or digital rotation.

In published reports evaluating manual or digital rotation, success rates are high, ranging from to 74% to 90%.[57,74–76] Full cervical dilation, maternal age less than 35, and multiparity were positively associated with successful rotation.[74,76] Conversely, nulliparity and maternal age greater than age 35, as well as Asian race/ethnicity, induction of labor and epidural use, labor dystocia as indication for rotation, and subsequent attempt after initial failure were associated with failure of manual rotation.[74,76] None of these studies observed an increase in adverse neonatal outcomes compared with expectant management, and in one study, a reduction in neonatal Apgar scores less than 7 at 5 minutes was associated with manual rotation.[57] Of the studies examining cesarean rate, severe perineal laceration (defined as anal sphincter involvement), postpartum hemorrhage, and chorioamnionitis were reduced with a practice of manual rotation, whereas increased rates of cervical laceration were associated with manual rotation in one study.[57,73]

In the event of failed manual rotation, or if expedited delivery is indicated, rotational forceps or forceps from the occiput posterior position may be considered. Although the number of skilled providers offering rotational forceps has decreased substantially in the last 50 years with the concurrent increase in cesarean delivery, there have been recent calls for increasing training opportunities citing the high rates of success with the procedure.[2,77] Recent publications including retrospective cohort studies and prospective observational studies suggest that rotational forceps with subsequent spontaneous or forceps-assisted delivery from occiput anterior when compared with forceps-assisted delivery from occiput posterior position resulted in reduced perineal trauma and did not result in significant increases in adverse neonatal outcomes.[78,79] Compared with cesarean delivery from the second stage, rotational forceps were associated with reduced rates of postpartum hemorrhage and reduced neonatal intensive care unit admissions.[80]

Vacuum-assisted vaginal delivery from the occiput posterior position may also be offered. Although associated with a lower rate of anal sphincter injury compared with forceps-assisted deliveries from occiput posterior, the success rate with vacuum-assisted delivery is generally lower than with forceps-assisted deliveries from both occiput posterior and anterior positions.[81] Given the concern for increased risk of neonatal trauma, including significant laceration as well as the high failure rate, rotational vacuum deliveries, particularly with rotation of greater than 45°, are discouraged by some professional societies.[82] Finally, cesarean delivery, particularly in the setting of labor dystocia and persistent occiput posterior or occiput transverse position, may be offered. As previously discussed, unintentional laceration and postpartum hemorrhage are greater at the time of cesarean delivery following prolonged second stage and in the setting of occiput posterior, so efforts should be made to improve vaginal delivery rates and, in the event of cesarean delivery, to anticipate these complications.

SUMMARY

Fetal malpresentation and malposition are commonly encountered in modern obstetrics and have considerable clinical consequences. Accurate identification of the fetal presentation and position is critical to appropriate management. Ultimately, the options available to patients are provider dependent and rely on an informed discussion of the risks and benefits. Appropriate comparison groups and future pregnancies should be considered when considering outcomes. As others have noted, making efforts to provide training opportunities to providers most likely to manage these challenging situations is necessary to continue optimizing and individualizing care for women and neonates.

REFERENCES

1. Caughey AB, Cahill AG, Guise JM, et al. Safe prevention of the primary cesarean delivery. Am J Obstet Gynecol 2014;210(3):179–93.
2. Barth WH Jr. Persistent occiput posterior. Obstet Gynecol 2015;125(3):695–709.

3. Demol S, Bashiri A, Furman B, et al. Breech presentation is a risk factor for intra-partum and neonatal death in preterm delivery. Eur J Obstet Gynecol Reprod Biol 2000;93(1):47–51.

4. Hickok DE, Gordon DC, Milberg JA, et al. The frequency of breech presentation by gestational age at birth: a large population-based study. Am J Obstet Gynecol 1992;166(3):851–2.

5. Martin JA, Hamilton BE, Osterman MJ, et al. Births: final data for 2015. Natl Vital Stat Rep 2017;66(1):1.

6. Ford JB, Roberts CL, Nassar N, et al. Recurrence of breech presentation in consecutive pregnancies. BJOG 2010;117(7):830–6.

7. Roberts CL, Algert CS, Peat B, et al. Small fetal size: a risk factor for breech birth at term. Int J Gynaecol Obstet 1999;67(1):1–8.

8. Sherer DM, Spong CY, Minior VK, et al. Increased incidence of fetal growth restriction in association with breech presentation in preterm deliveries <32 weeks. Am J Perinatol 1997;14(1):35–7.

9. Chou MR, Kreiser D, Taslimi MM, et al. Vaginal versus ultrasound examination of fetal occiput position during the second stage of labor. Am J Obstet Gynecol 2004;191(2):521–4.

10. Hua M, Odibo AO, Longman RE, et al. Congenital uterine anomalies and adverse pregnancy outcomes. Am J Obstet Gynecol 2011;205(6):558.e1-5.

11. Stout MJ, Odibo AO, Graseck AS, et al. Leiomyomas at routine second-trimester ultrasound examination and adverse obstetric outcomes. Obstet Gynecol 2010;116(5):1056–63.

12. Macharey G, Gissler M, Rahkonen L, et al. Breech presentation at term and associated obstetric risks factors-a nationwide population based cohort study. Arch Gynecol Obstet 2017;295(4):833–8.

13. Zsirai L, Csakany GM, Vargha P, et al. Breech presentation: its predictors and consequences. An analysis of the Hungarian Tauffer Obstetric Database (1996-2011). Acta Obstet Gynecol Scand 2016;95(3):347–54.

14. Pradhan P, Mohajer M, Deshpande S. Outcome of term breech births: 10-year experience at a district general hospital. BJOG 2005;112(2):218–22.

15. Rietberg CC, Elferink-Stinkens PM, Brand R, et al. Term breech presentation in the Netherlands from 1995 to 1999: mortality and morbidity in relation to the mode of delivery of 33824 infants. BJOG 2003;110(6):604–9.

16. Aisenbrey GA, Catanzarite VA, Nelson C. External cephalic version: predictors of success. Obstet Gynecol 1999;94(5 Pt 1):783–6.

17. Cluver C, Gyte GM, Sinclair M, et al. Interventions for helping to turn term breech babies to head first presentation when using external cephalic version. Cochrane Database Syst Rev 2015;(2):CD000184.

18. Kok M, Cnossen J, Gravendeel L, et al. Clinical factors to predict the outcome of external cephalic version: a metaanalysis. Am J Obstet Gynecol 2008;199(6):630.e1-7 [discussion: e1–5].

19. Goetzinger KR, Harper LM, Tuuli MG, et al. Effect of regional anesthesia on the success rate of external cephalic version: a systematic review and meta-analysis. Obstet Gynecol 2011;118(5):1137–44.

20. Magro-Malosso ER, Saccone G, Di Tommaso M, et al. Neuraxial analgesia to increase the success rate of external cephalic version: a systematic review and meta-analysis of randomized controlled trials. Am J Obstet Gynecol 2016;215(3):276–86.

21. Grootscholten K, Kok M, Oei SG, et al. External cephalic version-related risks: a meta-analysis. Obstet Gynecol 2008;112(5):1143–51.

22. Hannah ME, Hannah WJ, Hewson SA, et al. Planned caesarean section versus planned vaginal birth for breech presentation at term: a randomised multicentre trial. Term Breech Trial Collaborative Group. Lancet 2000;356(9239):1375–83.
23. Hannah ME, Whyte H, Hannah WJ, et al. Maternal outcomes at 2 years after planned cesarean section versus planned vaginal birth for breech presentation at term: the international randomized term breech trial. Am J Obstet Gynecol 2004;191(3):917–27.
24. Whyte H, Hannah ME, Saigal S, et al. Outcomes of children at 2 years after planned cesarean birth versus planned vaginal birth for breech presentation at term: the International Randomized Term Breech Trial. Am J Obstet Gynecol 2004;191(3):864–71.
25. Giuliani A, Scholl WM, Basver A, et al. Mode of delivery and outcome of 699 term singleton breech deliveries at a single center. Am J Obstet Gynecol 2002;187(6):1694–8.
26. Munstedt K, von Georgi R, Reucher S, et al. Term breech and long-term morbidity – cesarean section versus vaginal breech delivery. Eur J Obstet Gynecol Reprod Biol 2001;96(2):163–7.
27. Alarab M, Regan C, O'Connell MP, et al. Singleton vaginal breech delivery at term: still a safe option. Obstet Gynecol 2004;103(3):407–12.
28. Laros RK Jr, Flanagan TA, Kilpatrick SJ. Management of term breech presentation: a protocol of external cephalic version and selective trial of labor. Am J Obstet Gynecol 1995;172(6):1916–23 [discussion: 1923–5].
29. Gemer O, Segal S. Incidence and contribution of predisposing factors to transverse lie presentation. Int J Gynaecol Obstet 1994;44(3):219–21.
30. Hankins GD, Hammond TL, Snyder RR, et al. Transverse lie. Am J Perinatol 1990;7(1):66–70.
31. Uygur D, Kis S, Tuncer R, et al. Risk factors and infant outcomes associated with umbilical cord prolapse. Int J Gynaecol Obstet 2002;78(2):127–30.
32. Bashiri A, Burstein E, Bar-David J, et al. Face and brow presentation: independent risk factors. J Matern Fetal Neonatal Med 2008;21(6):357–60.
33. Shaffer BL, Cheng YW, Vargas JE, et al. Face presentation: predictors and delivery route. Am J Obstet Gynecol 2006;194(5):e10–12.
34. Gardberg M, Leonova Y, Laakkonen E. Malpresentations–impact on mode of delivery. Acta Obstet Gynecol Scand 2011;90(5):540–2.
35. Cheng YW, Caughey AB. Malpresentation and malposition. Management of labor and delivery. John Wiley & Sons, Ltd; 2015. p. 172–92.
36. Vialle R, Pietin-Vialle C, Ilharreborde B, et al. Spinal cord injuries at birth: a multicenter review of nine cases. J Matern Fetal Neonatal Med 2007;20(6):435–40.
37. Stitely ML, Gherman RB. Labor with abnormal presentation and position. Obstet Gynecol Clin North Am 2005;32(2):165–79.
38. Breen JL, Wiesmeier E. Compound presentation: a survey of 131 patients. Obstet Gynecol 1968;32(3):419–22.
39. Goplerud J, Eastman NJ. Compound presentation; a survey of 65 cases. Obstet Gynecol 1953;1(1):59–66.
40. Byrne H, Sleight S, Gordon A, et al. Unusual rectal trauma due to compound fetal presentation. J Obstet Gynaecol 2006;26(2):174–5.
41. Kwok CS, Judkins CL, Sherratt M. Forearm injury associated with compound presentation and prolonged labour. J Neonatal Surg 2015;4(3):40.
42. Tebes CC, Mehta P, Calhoun DA, et al. Congenital ischemic forearm necrosis associated with a compound presentation. J Matern Fetal Med 1999;8(5):231–3.

43. Cheng YW, Shaffer BL, Caughey AB. The association between persistent occiput posterior position and neonatal outcomes. Obstet Gynecol 2006;107(4):837–44.

44. Fitzpatrick M, McQuillan K, O'Herlihy C. Influence of persistent occiput posterior position on delivery outcome. Obstet Gynecol 2001;98(6):1027–31.

45. Sizer AR, Nirmal DM. Occipitoposterior position: associated factors and obstetric outcome in nulliparas. Obstet Gynecol 2000;96(5 Pt 1):749–52.

46. Lieberman E, Davidson K, Lee-Parritz A, et al. Changes in fetal position during labor and their association with epidural analgesia. Obstet Gynecol 2005; 105(5 Pt 1):974–82.

47. Gardberg M, Tuppurainen M. Persistent occiput posterior presentation–a clinical problem. Acta Obstet Gynecol Scand 1994;73(1):45–7.

48. Vitner D, Paltieli Y, Haberman S, et al. Prospective multicenter study of ultrasound-based measurements of fetal head station and position throughout labor. Ultrasound Obstet Gynecol 2015;46(5):611–5.

49. Sherer DM, Miodovnik M, Bradley KS, et al. Intrapartum fetal head position I: comparison between transvaginal digital examination and transabdominal ultrasound assessment during the active stage of labor. Ultrasound Obstet Gynecol 2002;19(3):258–63.

50. Sherer DM, Miodovnik M, Bradley KS, et al. Intrapartum fetal head position II: comparison between transvaginal digital examination and transabdominal ultrasound assessment during the second stage of labor. Ultrasound Obstet Gynecol 2002;19(3):264–8.

51. Ponkey SE, Cohen AP, Heffner LJ, et al. Persistent fetal occiput posterior position: obstetric outcomes. Obstet Gynecol 2003;101(5 Pt 1):915–20.

52. Ghi T, Youssef A, Martelli F, et al. Narrow subpubic arch angle is associated with higher risk of persistent occiput posterior position at delivery. Ultrasound Obstet Gynecol 2016;48(4):511–5.

53. Gardberg M, Stenwall O, Laakkonen E. Recurrent persistent occipito-posterior position in subsequent deliveries. BJOG 2004;111(2):170–1.

54. Anim-Somuah M, Smyth RM, Jones L. Epidural versus non-epidural or no analgesia in labour. Cochrane Database Syst Rev 2011;(12):CD000331.

55. Senecal J, Xiong X, Fraser WD. Effect of fetal position on second-stage duration and labor outcome. Obstet Gynecol 2005;105(4):763–72.

56. Cheng YW, Norwitz ER, Caughey AB. The relationship of fetal position and ethnicity with shoulder dystocia and birth injury. Am J Obstet Gynecol 2006; 195(3):856–62.

57. Shaffer BL, Cheng YW, Vargas JE, et al. Manual rotation to reduce caesarean delivery in persistent occiput posterior or transverse position. J Matern Fetal Neonatal Med 2011;24(1):65–72.

58. Gardberg M, Laakkonen E, Salevaara M. Intrapartum sonography and persistent occiput posterior position: a study of 408 deliveries. Obstet Gynecol 1998; 91(5 Pt 1):746–9.

59. de la Torre L, Gonzalez-Quintero VH, Mayor-Lynn K, et al. Significance of accidental extensions in the lower uterine segment during cesarean delivery. Am J Obstet Gynecol 2006;194(5):e4–6.

60. Sung JF, Daniels KI, Brodzinsky L, et al. Cesarean delivery outcomes after a prolonged second stage of labor. Am J Obstet Gynecol 2007;197(3):306.e1-5.

61. Akmal S, Tsoi E, Howard R, et al. Investigation of occiput posterior delivery by intrapartum sonography. Ultrasound Obstet Gynecol 2004;24(4):425–8.

62. Peregrine E, O'Brien P, Jauniaux E. Impact on delivery outcome of ultrasonographic fetal head position prior to induction of labor. Obstet Gynecol 2007; 109(3):618–25.

63. Shetty J, Aahir V, Pandey D, et al. Fetal head position during the first stage of labor: comparison between vaginal examination and transabdominal ultrasound. ISRN Obstet Gynecol 2014;2014:314617.

64. Akmal S, Kametas N, Tsoi E, et al. Comparison of transvaginal digital examination with intrapartum sonography to determine fetal head position before instrumental delivery. Ultrasound Obstet Gynecol 2003;21(5):437–40.

65. Ramphul M, Kennelly M, Murphy DJ. Establishing the accuracy and acceptability of abdominal ultrasound to define the foetal head position in the second stage of labour: a validation study. Eur J Obstet Gynecol Reprod Biol 2012;164(1):35–9.

66. Zahalka N, Sadan O, Malinger G, et al. Comparison of transvaginal sonography with digital examination and transabdominal sonography for the determination of fetal head position in the second stage of labor. Am J Obstet Gynecol 2005; 193(2):381–6.

67. Guittier MJ, Othenin-Girard V, de Gasquet B, et al. Maternal positioning to correct occiput posterior fetal position during the first stage of labour: a randomised controlled trial. BJOG 2016;123(13):2199–207.

68. Hunter S, Hofmeyr GJ, Kulier R. Hands and knees posture in late pregnancy or labour for fetal malposition (lateral or posterior). Cochrane Database Syst Rev 2007;(4):CD001063.

69. Stremler R, Hodnett E, Petryshen P, et al. Randomized controlled trial of hands-and-knees positioning for occipitoposterior position in labor. Birth 2005;32(4): 243–51.

70. Kariminia A, Chamberlain ME, Keogh J, et al. Randomised controlled trial of effect of hands and knees posturing on incidence of occiput posterior position at birth. BMJ 2004;328(7438):490.

71. Desbriere R, Blanc J, Le Du R, et al. Is maternal posturing during labor efficient in preventing persistent occiput posterior position? A randomized controlled trial. Am J Obstet Gynecol 2013;208(1):60.e1-8.

72. Le Ray C, Lepleux F, De La Calle A, et al. Lateral asymmetric decubitus position for the rotation of occipito-posterior positions: multicenter randomized controlled trial EVADELA. Am J Obstet Gynecol 2016;215(4):511.e1-7.

73. Le Ray C, Deneux-Tharaux C, Khireddine I, et al. Manual rotation to decrease operative delivery in posterior or transverse positions. Obstet Gynecol 2013; 122(3):634–40.

74. Le Ray C, Serres P, Schmitz T, et al. Manual rotation in occiput posterior or transverse positions: risk factors and consequences on the cesarean delivery rate. Obstet Gynecol 2007;110(4):873–9.

75. Reichman O, Gdansky E, Latinsky B, et al. Digital rotation from occipito-posterior to occipito-anterior decreases the need for cesarean section. Eur J Obstet Gynecol Reprod Biol 2008;136(1):25–8.

76. Shaffer BL, Cheng YW, Vargas JE, et al. Manual rotation of the fetal occiput: predictors of success and delivery. Am J Obstet Gynecol 2006;194(5):e7–9.

77. Tempest N, Hart A, Walkinshaw S, et al. A re-evaluation of the role of rotational forceps: retrospective comparison of maternal and perinatal outcomes following different methods of birth for malposition in the second stage of labour. BJOG 2013;120(10):1277–84.

78. Benavides L, Wu JM, Hundley AF, et al. The impact of occiput posterior fetal head position on the risk of anal sphincter injury in forceps-assisted vaginal deliveries. Am J Obstet Gynecol 2005;192(5):1702–6.
79. Bradley MS, Kaminski RJ, Streitman DC, et al. Effect of rotation on perineal lacerations in forceps-assisted vaginal deliveries. Obstet Gynecol 2013;122(1):132–7.
80. Stock SJ, Josephs K, Farquharson S, et al. Maternal and neonatal outcomes of successful Kielland's rotational forceps delivery. Obstet Gynecol 2013;121(5):1032–9.
81. Damron DP, Capeless EL. Operative vaginal delivery: a comparison of forceps and vacuum for success rate and risk of rectal sphincter injury. Am J Obstet Gynecol 2004;191(3):907–10.
82. Cargill YM, MacKinnon CJ, Arsenault MY, et al. Guidelines for operative vaginal birth. J Obstet Gynaecol Can 2004;26(8):747–61.

Labor and Delivery of Twin Pregnancies

Stephanie Melka, MD, James Miller, MD, Nathan S. Fox, MD*

KEYWORDS

- Twins • Labor • Delivery • Breech extraction • Active management • Cesarean

KEY POINTS

- In twin pregnancies, planned vaginal delivery is not associated with adverse maternal or neonatal outcomes, compared with planned cesarean delivery, assuming the obstetrician is experienced in twin delivery.
- Active management of the second stage of labor consists of breech extraction of the non-vertex second twin and internal podalic version and breech extraction of the unengaged vertex second twin.
- Active management of the second stage of labor achieves a high rate of vaginal deliveries and very low rates of combined vaginal-cesarean delivery.

INTRODUCTION

The incidence of twin pregnancies in the United States has increased over the past few decades, and twins now represent 3.4% of all US live births.[1] In the United States, approximately 75% of twins are delivered by cesarean delivery (CD).[2] Reasons for the high CD rate in the United States include malpresentation of the first or second twin, prematurity, maternal comorbidities, and patient preference. However, recent literature suggests that, for many women with twin pregnancies, vaginal delivery can be achieved without increasing maternal or neonatal morbidity. This article reviews the management of labor in twin pregnancies.

BACKGROUND

Mode of Delivery and Success Rates of Twin Vaginal Delivery

Overall, the goal of a twin delivery is to provide a safe delivery for the mother and both babies. With regard to mode of delivery, there are 3 potential outcomes:

Disclosure: The authors have nothing to disclose.
Maternal Fetal Medicine Associates, PLLC, and The Department of Obstetrics, Gynecology, and Reproductive Science, Icahn School of Medicine at Mount Sinai, 70 East 90th Street, New York, NY 10128, USA
* Corresponding author.
E-mail address: nfox@mfmnyc.com

Obstet Gynecol Clin N Am 44 (2017) 645–654
http://dx.doi.org/10.1016/j.ogc.2017.08.004
0889-8545/17/© 2017 Elsevier Inc. All rights reserved.

- Vaginal delivery of both twins
- CD of both twins
- Vaginal delivery of twin A followed by CD of twin B (combined vaginal-CD)

In general, vaginal delivery of both twins is the most desirable outcome (discussed later) because neonatal outcomes are similar regardless of mode of delivery and because it avoids the maternal morbidity associated with CD for the current pregnancy and future pregnancies. CD of both twins is the next desirable outcome. The least desirable outcome is a combined vaginal-CD. This type of delivery adds the morbidities of labor, vaginal delivery, and CD. It also frequently is associated with a complication between the delivery of the first and second twin.

Rates for the 3 modes of delivery vary in the literature. In the United States, the overall rate of CD for twins is approximately 75%[2] and up to 10% of women who deliver the first twin vaginally have an unplanned CD of the second twin.[3] In Ireland, the CD rate for twins is 65% (23% for women who labored) with a 3% rate of combined vaginal-CD.[4] A study from France of 657 women with twin pregnancies attempting labor showed a CD rate of 21.1% with a combined vaginal-CD rate of only 0.5%.[5]

The different CD rates and different combined vaginal-CD rates are mostly caused by differences in management of a nonvertex second twin. In the United States, malpresentation of the second twin is often the reason for CD because most modern-trained obstetricians lack the knowledge and experience to perform a breech delivery. However, in France, where the success rates were best, the obstetricians were comfortable with delivery of the second twin regardless of presentation because they routinely used active management of the second stage of labor, which consists of 2 essential tools: breech extraction of the nonvertex second twin and internal podalic version and breech extraction of the unengaged vertex second twin. Studies in the United States are consistent with these approaches. For example, among 130 women with twin pregnancies attempting labor, the CD rate was 15.4% with 0% having a combined vaginal-CD.[6] In a follow-up study of 286 women with twin pregnancies attempting vaginal delivery, these rates were 17.8% and 0%, respectively.[7]

Active management of the second stage in a twin gestation is used to deliver the second twin by breech extraction in all cases except when the second twin is in an engaged vertex presentation. If there are no contraindications to vaginal delivery, patients with twin pregnancies who labor and have active management of the second stage should expect high rates of vaginal deliveries and very low rates of combined vaginal-CD.[5,6] Both retrospective studies showed similar short-term neonatal outcomes for twins, regardless of planned mode of delivery.[5,6]

Mode of Delivery: Safety of Vaginal Twin Delivery

Most older studies examining the safest mode of delivery for twins were retrospective and compared either twins born vaginally with twins born by CD, or compared twins with planned vaginal delivery with twins with planned CD. The conclusions of those studies were mixed,[5,6,8–11] with some finding benefit to CD and others finding no difference in outcomes. However, the retrospective studies all contain significant selection bias, and it is difficult to make any definitive conclusions from these types of analyses.

The Twin Birth Study was a prospective, randomized trial of planned vaginal delivery versus planned CD for twin pregnancies, and the results were published in 2013.[12]

This multicenter study from 2003 to 2011 across 106 centers in 25 countries included 2804 women with twin pregnancies 32 0/7 to 38 6/7 weeks who were randomized to planned vaginal delivery versus planned CD. Inclusion criteria included estimated fetal weights 1500g to 4000g; the first twin had to be in vertex presentation; both twins had to be alive, and there were no other contraindications to labor. Both dichorionic and monochorionic twins were included, but monoamniotic twins were excluded. The primary outcome was a composite of fetal and neonatal mortality or serious neonatal morbidity at 28 days of life, and did not differ significantly between the two groups (2.2% in the planned CD group vs 1.9% in the planned vaginal delivery group; $P = .49$). There were no differences in any secondary outcomes between the groups, including individual fetal or neonatal outcomes, and maternal composite morbidity. Also, the primary outcome was not affected by position of the second twin, gestational age, chorionicity, maternal age, or perinatal mortality in the country of residence. Follow-up examination of the children at 2 years of life did not show any differences in neurodevelopmental outcomes between the groups.[13] Maternal outcomes also did not differ at 3 months after delivery.[14] Based on the results of this randomized trial, for women with a twin pregnancy greater than 32 weeks with the first twin in vertex presentation, planned CD is not associated with any known improvement in maternal or neonatal morbidity or mortality.

In the Twin Birth Study, among the 1393 women in the planned vaginal delivery group, the CD rate was 39.6% and the combined vaginal-CD rate was 4.2%. After removing the 196 women who had their CD before labor, for the women who attempted labor, the CD rate was 34.4% (412 out of 1197) and the combined vaginal-CD rate was 4.9% (57 out of 1197). All delivering obstetricians were reported to be experienced at vaginal twin delivery, but no specific details were reported regarding expertise in breech extraction or internal podalic version.

Mode of Delivery: Conclusion

Patients with twin pregnancies greater than 32 weeks with the first twin in vertex presentation should be counseled that planned vaginal delivery is not associated with adverse maternal or neonatal outcomes, compared with planned CD, assuming the obstetrician is experienced in twin delivery. If the mother does attempt labor, the likelihood of a vaginal delivery is approximately 65% to 75% and the likelihood of a combined vaginal-CD is approximately 3% to 10%. However, if the delivering obstetrician is comfortable with active management of the second stage, including breech extraction and internal podalic version, the likelihood of vaginal delivery can be as high as 85% and the combined vaginal-CD rate could be less than 1%. Planned vaginal delivery of twins is currently encouraged in well-selected patients.[15]

PROTOCOL FOR DELIVERY OF TWINS

The approach to vaginal delivery of twins usually involves institutional guidelines about selection and management. There are no specific approaches that have been well studied compared with others. Thus, this article presents an example of a specific protocol for the delivery of twin pregnancies. This protocol has several components.

Patient Selection

Not all women with twin pregnancies should attempt a trial of labor. First, the patient should desire a vaginal delivery and there should be no other contraindications to vaginal delivery. In addition, the following is required:

- Twin A must be in vertex presentation.
- Twin B's estimated fetal weight should be greater than 1500g.[a]
- If the estimated fetal weight of twin B is greater than twin A, the discordance should be less than 20%.[a]

Third-Trimester Counseling

All patients with twin pregnancies considering vaginal delivery are counseled in the third trimester, including:

- A devoted counseling session with a delivering obstetrician
- An opportunity to accept or decline an attempt at vaginal delivery
- Detailed documentation in the prenatal record

Timing of Delivery

Because of the increased risk of intrauterine fetal demise in twin pregnancies, uncomplicated twin pregnancies are delivered earlier than singletons. Delivery is commonly recommended for twin pregnancies at the following gestational ages, or sooner if other indications are present[16]

- Dichorionic diamniotic twins: 38 weeks
- Monochorionic diamniotic twins: 37 weeks

These recommendations are made to balance the increasing risk of stillbirth and the decreasing risk of prematurity as a pregnancy progresses, as well as the small risks of early term deliveries.

Induction of Labor

When a woman with a twin pregnancy has an indication for delivery, or she has reached the gestational age at which delivery is recommended, induction of labor is offered as an option.

Twin pregnancies can use the same approaches as singleton gestations; for example, cervical ripening with prostaglandins or a transcervical Foley balloon catheter.

Induction of labor has similar success in twin pregnancies as in singleton pregnancies, and the risk factors for failed induction are the same (nulliparity, advanced maternal age, low Bishop score).[17] For example, in one study, for women with twins undergoing induction of labor, nulliparous women had a 27.9% likelihood of CD, whereas multiparous women had a 5.1% likelihood of CD.[17]

Regional Anesthesia

For all women with twin pregnancies attempting labor, regional anesthesia (epidural) is recommended for several reasons:

- In the event of an unplanned CD in labor. Trying to place an epidural in this setting could be difficult in a woman with twins and general anesthesia carries an increased risk of aspiration.

---

[a] If twin B is in vertex presentation, then the estimated fetal weight criteria for twin B listed earlier do not apply. The criteria are meant to decrease the risk of head entrapment. Head entrapment at the cervix is thought to be more common in preterm babies in whom the head circumference is larger than the abdominal circumference or in deliveries in which twin B is significantly larger than twin A. However, data supporting this concern are limited. Patients in this scenario must be counseled that they are at increased risk for combined vaginal-CD because they would not be candidates for breech extraction.

- Maternal comfort can facilitate easier fetal monitoring of both twins.
- Most importantly, to allow for breech extraction of the second twin. Breech extraction cannot be easily performed without anesthesia.

Management of Labor

Most labor management for twins is similar to that for a singleton gestation. Patients are given a clear liquid diet, and intravenous fluids are administered at a maintenance rate (typically 125 mL/h). Continuous external fetal heart rate monitoring is performed for both twins until delivery. Because monitoring both twins externally can be technically challenging, placement of an internal scalp electrode for twin A can be performed as needed, leaving only twin B with external monitoring. If continuous fetal heart rate monitoring cannot be achieved, CD is recommended.

Assessment of the labor curve and appropriate progress in labor does not differ for twin pregnancies compared with singleton pregnancies. Obstetric interventions in labor and the decision to perform a CD for arrest of labor or nonreassuring fetal heart rate are according to the same indications as in singleton pregnancies.

During labor, the patient remains in a standard labor room until the cervix is fully dilated, at which point she is transferred to the operating room for delivery. Consideration should be given to delivering all twins in the operating room for several reasons:

- The operating room is the largest room on labor and delivery, which allows space for all personnel present for delivery.
- The overhead lighting allows for better visualization.
- Decreased time to delivery if an emergent CD is warranted.

For all twin deliveries, the following personnel are present in the operating room:

- Two obstetricians (ideally one of whom is a learner, such as a resident or junior attending).
- Two pediatric teams, 1 for each twin.
- Three nurses: – 1 for the patient and 1 for each twin.
- A surgical technician, in the event of a CD, or to assist with instruments needed for vaginal delivery.
- An anesthesiologist.

The patient pushes in the second stage in the operating room using foot rests attached to the operating room table and using a large foam wedge behind her to allow her to be sitting at a 45° angle. Her partner is encouraged to be with her, similar to a singleton vaginal delivery. Continuous fetal heart rate monitoring is maintained for both twins during the second stage of labor.

All personnel in the operating room wear surgical scrubs, masks, and head covers, but no one aside from the surgical technician is scrubbed at this time.

Delivery: Active Management of the Second Stage

The delivery of twin A proceeds as a standard singleton vertex delivery, with the use of operative delivery and episiotomy as indicated. After the first twin delivers, the cord is clamped twice with small plastic cord clamps and cut and twin A is handed to the mother or the awaiting pediatricians. A single clamp is left on the cord of twin A (to help differentiate the 2 placentas after birth).

After delivery of the first twin is complete, a vaginal examination is done to determine the presenting part of twin B and the mode of delivery for the second twin.

Twin B: cephalic and engaged

If twin B is cephalic and engaged in the maternal pelvis, continuous fetal heart rate monitoring is continued until delivery and the mother begins to push again. Frequently, oxytocin needs to be given (or the rate increased) to maintain a regular contraction pattern. As maternal contractions bring the fetal head further into the pelvis, artificial rupture of membranes is performed with maternal expulsive efforts to facilitate delivery. Operative delivery and episiotomy are performed for the usual indications.

Twin B: breech or transverse

If twin B is in breech or transverse presentation, a total breech extraction is performed. This extraction should occur within several minutes of delivery for twin A. Delivering twin B before the cervix contracts decreases the likelihood of a head entrapment in the cervical canal.

To perform breech extraction, the fetal feet are grasped at the ankles and pulled caudally, maintaining a good hold because the membranes typically rupture at this time. If not, artificial rupture of membranes is performed. If both feet cannot be grasped, it is appropriate to pull on 1 foot until the foot reaches past the introitus, at which point the second leg and foot can usually be identified and delivered.

As the breech delivers past the introitus, the umbilical cord is lengthened and the infant is grasped with 1 hand on each hip. The operator's thumbs should be placed on the sacrum and the hands wrapped around the sides and grasping the front of the infant with the index fingers on the anterior superior iliac spines. Pressure higher or more lateral on the back could cause trauma to the kidneys or adrenal glands. Pulling caudally delivers the fetal abdomen and chest, with concurrent 180° clockwise and counterclockwise rotation to dislodge a possible nuchal arm, as needed. As the fetal scapulae come into view, the arms are then delivered. If the right scapula is visible, the provider's right hand is used and the right thumb is placed on the right scapula, and the fingers are used to sweep the right arm in a down-and-out fashion. The infant is then rotated clockwise, and the left arm is delivered in the same fashion with the operator's left hand.

The head is delivered by performing the Mauriceau-Smellie-Veit maneuver. The first and middle fingers of the obstetrician's dominant hand are placed on the fetal mandible on each side of the fetal mouth with the palm on the baby's chest. The nondominant hand is placed along the upper back with the middle finger on the occiput. By pulling down on the maxillae and pushing down on the occiput, this maintains flexion of the fetal head. An assistant can also provide suprapubic pressure to aid with flexion of the head. As the body is elevated, the head is then delivered through the vagina. If further fetal head flexion is needed, Piper forceps can be used.

Twin B: Unengaged

If twin B is vertex or oblique, but unengaged, there is an option for an internal podalic version of twin B. To perform this maneuver, one hand is placed in the vagina and the other on the maternal abdomen. The hand in the vagina should be the one opposite the side of the fetal back. So, if the fetal back is to the maternal right, the operator's right hand is placed in the vagina and the left hand on the maternal abdomen. The operator's internal hand first elevates the vertex higher into the uterine cavity and then reaches for a fetal foot. The outer hand then continues to elevate the vertex, while the internal hand pulls the feet caudally, rotating the baby to complete breech presentation. Delivery then proceeds as a breech extraction, as described earlier.

After delivery of the second twin, the umbilical cord is clamped and cut and then marked as twin B with 2 clamps. The baby is handed to the mother or the second team of pediatricians. Cord blood gases are obtained and the placentas are then delivered. Oxytocin is administered, as well as any additional uterotonics as needed. Any lacerations are repaired and the patient is returned to the supine position.

TWIN DELIVERY: COMPLICATIONS AND MANAGEMENT

Twin pregnancies are at increased risk for delivery complications relative to singleton pregnancies. There is an increased risk for uterine atony, postpartum hemorrhage, and difficult extraction. There are also potential complications associated with active management of the second stage, such as cord prolapse, hand presentation, nuchal arm, and head entrapment. With proper patient selection and provider training, most of these complications can be prevented or mitigated to achieve a safe delivery. Some of the most common complications and their management are listed here.

Uterine Atony

An enlarged uterus (overdistended by twins) is a known risk factor for uterine atony and postpartum hemorrhage. On admission to the hospital, a sample of blood should be sent to the blood bank to crossmatch at least 2 units of packed red blood cells for all twin deliveries. After delivery, routine active management of the third stage of labor (uterine massage and intravenous oxytocin) should be used and there should be a low threshold to administer any additional uterotonic agents.

Difficult Extraction

Regardless of mode of delivery, extraction of twins can sometimes be a challenge. Occasionally, it can be difficult during CD to deliver twin A in vertex presentation. If an unengaged (floating) vertex is noted at the time of CD, twin B can be delivered first, instrumental delivery with vacuum or forceps can be used for twin A, or an attempt can be made to deliver twin A as a breech presentation. The pediatric team is present in the delivery room for all twin deliveries in case neonatal support or resuscitation is needed.

Unengaged Vertex of Twin B

If twin B is unengaged and vertex and given time to descend, there is a risk that the cord or fetal hand could descend below the vertex while it is unengaged. A CD is required in this setting because it is unsafe to perform an operative delivery with an unengaged vertex and unsafe to perform breech extraction because of the risk of head entrapment if too much time has elapsed after delivery of twin A.

Complications of Active Management During the Second Stage

Uterine hypertonicity
After delivery of twin A, the uterus may contract rapidly on twin B. In cases of malpresentation, it can be difficult to perform the necessary maneuvers to rotate and deliver the second twin in this setting. A single dose of nitroglycerin (100 μg intravenously given by the anesthesiologist) or a dose of terbutaline (250 μg given subcutaneously) can be used to relax a hypertonic uterus.

Malpresentation
In experienced hands, internal podalic version and breech extraction are used.

Failed breech extraction

If an attempt is made at breech extraction of twin B and it proves difficult, the obstetrician must know when to abandon the procedure and proceed with CD for twin B (combined vaginal-CD). In general, most internal podalic versions and breech extractions are performed within a few minutes of birth of twin A. If breech extraction of twin B has not been achieved after 5 minutes, staff should be notified to prepare for CD and an assistant should begin scrubbing. Maneuvers to achieve breech extraction should continue while final preparations are being made. In addition, CD should be started after 8 to 10 minutes have passed from the birth of twin A. The provider must consider whether it would be appropriate to use a midtransverse or classic incision rather than a low transverse incision depending on the clinical setting and maternal anatomy (fetal lie, distended bladder, length of second stage, and so forth).

Cord prolapse/hand presentation/funic presentation

Each of these conditions may be diagnosed after twin A has delivered. Internal podalic version and breech extraction of twin B can be performed promptly, avoiding the need for CD.

Nuchal arm

This condition occurs when the fetal arm is behind the fetal head and neck during breech extraction. It is relieved with rotation of the fetal body. For example, as twin B delivers, the sacrum is oriented anteriorly. If the left arm is reaching up and around behind the fetal head toward the fetal right shoulder (ie, the left arm is between the fetal head and the maternal bladder/anterior uterine wall), the fetal body should be rotated clockwise until the arm passes in front of the head, and then is delivered in standard fashion. A right nuchal arm is relieved with counterclockwise rotation of the fetal body. Another way to remember this is whichever arm is nuchal, that shoulder needs to rotate toward 12 o'clock (like windshield wipers).

Head entrapment

Head entrapment refers to the inability to deliver the fetal head during a breech extraction because it cannot pass through a contracted cervix. This situation is most likely to occur:

1. When twin B is significantly larger than twin A
2. In certain cases of prematurity (caused by the larger ratio of head to abdominal circumference)
3. When breech delivery is not performed in a prompt fashion

As the cervix contracts, the fetal abdomen and thorax can pass through, but the cervix prevents delivery of the fetal head. There are several maneuvers to assist with fetal head entrapment. The anesthesiologist should ensure the patient has good pain relief and administer a rapid-acting uterine relaxant. The assistant should provide suprapubic pressure, which flexes the fetal head and may assist in delivery. Duhrssen incisions can be made on the cervix using bandage scissors, incising at 2, 6, and 10 o'clock. This technique increases the diameter of the cervix, allowing the fetal head to pass through. If unsuccessful, CD is required.

SUMMARY

Obstetricians who care for twin pregnancies should be aware of the challenges that may arise during the labor and delivery. With recognition of these issues and proper training, providers should be able to help women with twin pregnancies achieve a safe delivery for them and their babies. With the use of breech extraction of the second twin and active management of the second stage of labor, women with twin pregnancies can also achieve a high vaginal delivery rate of both twins.

REFERENCES

1. Martin JA, Hamilton BE, Osterman MJ, et al. Births: final data for 2015. Natl Vital Stat Rep 2017;66(1):1.
2. Bateni ZH, Clark SL, Sangi-Haghpeykar H, et al. Trends in the delivery route of twin pregnancies in the United States, 2006-2013. Eur J Obstet Gynecol Reprod Biol 2016;205:120–6.
3. Wen SW, Fung KF, Oppenheimer L, et al. Occurrence and predictors of cesarean delivery for the second twin after vaginal delivery of the first twin. Obstet Gynecol 2004;103(3):413–9.
4. Breathnach FM, McAuliffe FM, Geary M, et al, Perinatal Ireland Research Consortium. Prediction of safe and successful vaginal twin birth. Am J Obstet Gynecol 2011;205(3):237.e1-7.
5. Schmitz T, Carnavalet Cde C, Azria E, et al. Neonatal outcomes of twin pregnancy according to the planned mode of delivery. Obstet Gynecol 2008;111(3): 695–703.
6. Fox NS, Silverstein M, Bender S, et al. Active second-stage management in twin pregnancies undergoing planned vaginal delivery in a U.S. population. Obstet Gynecol 2010;115(2 Pt 1):229–33.
7. Fox NS, Gupta S, Melka S, et al. Risk factors for cesarean delivery in twin pregnancies attempting vaginal delivery. Am J Obstet Gynecol 2015;212(1):106.e1-5.
8. Smith GC, Shah I, White IR, et al. Mode of delivery and the risk of delivery-related perinatal death among twins at term: a retrospective cohort study of 8073 births. BJOG 2005;112(8):1139–44.
9. Armson BA, O'Connell C, Persad V, et al. Determinants of perinatal mortality and serious neonatal morbidity in the second twin. Obstet Gynecol 2006;108(3 Pt 1): 556–64.
10. Yang Q, Wen SW, Chen Y, et al. Neonatal mortality and morbidity in vertex-vertex second twins according to mode of delivery and birth weight. J Perinatol 2006; 26(1):3–10.
11. Haest KM, Roumen FJ, Nijhuis JG. Neonatal and maternal outcomes in twin gestations > or =32 weeks according to the planned mode of delivery. Eur J Obstet Gynecol Reprod Biol 2005;123(1):17–21.
12. Barrett JF, Hannah ME, Hutton EK, et al, Twin Birth Study Collaborative Group. A randomized trial of planned cesarean or vaginal delivery for twin pregnancy. N Engl J Med 2013;369(14):1295–305.
13. Asztalos EV, Hannah ME, Hutton EK, et al. Twin birth study: 2-year neurodevelopmental follow-up of the randomized trial of planned cesarean or planned vaginal delivery for twin pregnancy. Am J Obstet Gynecol 2016;214(3):371.e1-19.
14. Hutton EK, Hannah ME, Ross S, et al, Twin Birth Study Collaborative Group. Maternal outcomes at 3 months after planned caesarean section versus planned vaginal birth for twin pregnancies in the twin birth study: a randomised controlled trial. BJOG 2015;122(12):1653–62.
15. Spong CY, Berghella V, Wenstrom KD, et al. Preventing the first cesarean delivery: summary of a joint Eunice Kennedy Shriver National Institute of Child Health and Human Development, Society for Maternal-Fetal Medicine, and American

College of Obstetricians and Gynecologists workshop. Obstet Gynecol 2012;
120(5):1181–93.

16. American College of Obstetricians and Gynecologists. ACOG committee opinion
no. 560: medically indicated late-preterm and early-term deliveries. Obstet Gynecol 2013;121(4):908–10.

17. Taylor M, Rebarber A, Saltzman DH, et al. Induction of labor in twin compared
with singleton pregnancies. Obstet Gynecol 2012;120(2 Pt 1):297–301.

Vaginal Birth After Cesarean Trends
Which Way Is the Pendulum Swinging?

James Sargent, MD*, Aaron B. Caughey, MD, PhD

KEYWORDS

- Cesarean • Labor and delivery • TOLAC • VBAC

KEY POINTS

- Cesarean delivery is associated with increased maternal and fetal risks that increase with each subsequent cesarean, potentially threatening future childbearing decisions.
- The US cesarean delivery rate has plateaued at 32% and currently less than 25% of women with a previous cesarean attempt a future trial of labor after cesarean (TOLAC).
- A TOLAC is associated with decreased maternal mortality, hysterectomy, and fever, but increased risk of uterine rupture, transfusion, neonatal encephalopathy, and perinatal mortality.
- Access to TOLAC is limited by resource availability, malpractice concerns, and provider failure to adequately counsel women regarding their choices.
- Future studies are needed to identify and address barriers to TOLAC availability.

INTRODUCTION

Cesarean deliveries (CDs) occur in one-third of all births in the United States[1] and, compared with vaginal deliveries, are associated with increased maternal and neonatal morbidity.[2–5] Additional CDs are associated with increased risk of abnormal placentation, intraoperative injury, massive transfusion, unplanned hysterectomy, and prolonged hospital stay,[6] underscoring the importance of reducing the incidence of CD when safely possible. Vaginal birth after cesarean (VBAC) can mitigate the high CD rate and associated complications, but the availability of a trial of labor after cesarean (TOLAC) has varied over time. This article outlines the factors influencing VBAC trends in addition to discussing the maternal and neonatal outcomes associated with TOLAC, specifically in certain high-risk populations.

Disclosure: The authors have no commercial or financial disclosures or conflicts of interest.
Department of Obstetrics and Gynecology, Oregon Health & Science University, 3181 Southwest Sam Jackson Park Road, L466, Portland, OR 97239-3098, USA
* Corresponding author.
E-mail address: sargenja@ohsu.edu

The Rise and Fall of Trial of Labor After Cesarean

In 1916, Edward Cragin,[7] in an address to the New York Association of Obstetricians and Gynecologists, coined the phrase "once a cesarean, always a cesarean," reflecting the dominant clinical philosophy of the time. In 1951, 2 reports outlining VBAC outcomes were published,[8,9] but the practice of a TOLAC did not receive much attention until the 1981 National Institutes of Health Consensus on Childbirth.[10] That report addressed the increasing rate of CD and focused on TOLAC as a means to decrease this national trend.[10,11] In 1988, the American College of Obstetricians and Gynecologists (ACOG) published guidelines for the safe practice of TOLAC and national rates of VBAC increased from 3% in 1981 to an all-time high of 28% in 1996,[12,13] whereas the CD rate simultaneously reached a nadir of 21%.[1]

In 1996, a large retrospective study was published comparing outcomes following TOLAC versus repeat CD in women with a previous CD and found an increase in major maternal complications in the TOLAC group (adjusted odds ratio [aOR], 1.8; 95% confidence interval [CI], 1.1–3.0) driven by the increased rate of uterine rupture (aOR, 5.2; 95% CI, 0.6–45.4).[14] There were no differences in minor maternal complications or neonatal outcomes with either mode of delivery. That study highlighted the increased risks of a failed TOLAC, which was reflected in the 1999 ACOG guidelines on VBAC.[11] Following that report, the rates of TOLAC and VBAC steadily declined to 16% and 9%, respectively, in 2006.[11,15] Concurrently, the CD rate increased annually until peaking at 33% in 2009 and subsequently plateaued over the past 3 years at 32%.[1]

Much of the decline in TOLAC was secondary to a provider-driven decrease in availability influenced by 2 changes in the 1999 ACOG VBAC guidelines.[11] The first modification was to recommend obstetricians to offer a TOLAC to eligible women rather than encourage one. The second modification was to require that surgical and anesthesia resources be immediately available for an emergency CD in the setting of a suspected uterine rupture. Following this, TOLAC availability declined because approximately one-third of hospitals and half of obstetric clinicians were either unable to meet the standard of being immediately available or were unwilling to risk subsequent litigation.[10] In the 2010 ACOG practice bulletin on VBAC, the investigators acknowledged that "[reports of uterine rupture], and the professional liability pressures they engendered, have resulted in a reversal of VBAC and [CD] trends,"[16] and that "concerns over liability have a major impact on the willingness of physicians and healthcare institutions to offer TOL [trial of labor]."[10,16] The decline in TOLAC has continued, with recent surveys of institutional TOLAC availability in California[17] and New Mexico[18] noting that only 57% and 41%, respectively, of responding institutions offered TOLAC in 2012.[17,18] Both studies found that the most common reasons for hospitals not offering TOLAC was the lack of obstetrician or anesthesia availability, in addition to the malpractice cost.

The Impact of Litigation Concerns

The fear of litigation greatly contributes to provider reticence when offering TOLAC.[19] The most common cause of malpractice litigation surrounding TOLAC is severe neonatal neurologic impairment following uterine rupture.[19] In these cases, the award, by jury verdict, can be substantial and cases are often settled even if the standard of care was met.[19] The 2009 ACOG Survey on Professional Liability revealed that 26% of responding ACOG members stopped offering TOLAC in the previous 3 years, with 20% reporting malpractice affordability or availability as the reason.[20] In response, the 2010 ACOG Practice Bulletin on VBAC stated, "restricting [TOLAC] access was not the intention of the College's past recommendations."[16] Instead, they qualified previous remarks stating, "the decision to offer and pursue TOLAC in a setting in which the option of immediate cesarean delivery is more limited should be carefully considered by patients and their healthcare provider."[16] The statement recognized that "respect for patient autonomy supports the concept that patients should be allowed to accept increased levels of risk, however, patients should be clearly informed of such potential increase in risk and management alternatives."[16]

Before undertaking a TOL, thorough documentation of informed consent is important to preserve patient autonomy, improve interprovider communication, and for liability protection. This process involves a discussion between the woman and her provider regarding the maternal and fetal risks in addition to the benefits of either a TOL or a repeat CD. Standardized consent forms can be used if they contain patient-specific information, including maternal and fetal factors that influence a patient's chance for a successful TOL or risk of uterine rupture. It should be emphasized to the patient that she may opt for a repeat CD at any time intrapartum. Such consent forms should, at a minimum, be completed during the antepartum or intrapartum period.[19]

Of note, a signed form does not always equate to informed consent; it does not ensure comprehension of a patient's choices or liability protection for the physician. One group of investigators found that, in a previously counseled population, there were critical knowledge gaps between the patient-perceived likelihood of TOLAC success and risks of TOLAC versus repeat CD, with 45% to 73% of patients replying, "I do not know" to pertinent questions.[21] To avoid lack of comprehension, an ongoing conversation throughout pregnancy must be undertaken with an emphasis on the patient's individual risks, chances for success, and the potential outcomes for each intended mode of delivery.

MODE OF DELIVERY OUTCOMES

The counseling process for TOL versus repeat CD depends on a thorough understanding of the risks and benefits of both options. The woman and her physician must decide between the risk of a repeat CD and that of a TOL. A repeat CD is associated with an increased possibility of maternal complications and can adversely affect future pregnancies. The risk of a TOL depends first on whether the TOL leads to a vaginal delivery versus a cesarean in labor. A TOL has improved maternal and neonatal outcomes compared with a repeat CD if successful, but has increased risk of maternal and neonatal morbidity and mortality in the setting of an unscheduled CD. Further, although both of these management approaches are considered safe, they each carry the risk of rare, serious complications (**Table 1**).

Maternal Outcomes

Maternal mortality
Since 2003, the overall maternal mortality in the United States has been 12 to 15 per 100,000 pregnancies, and for uncomplicated women with a history of CD the rate is slightly lower at 10 per 100,000 pregnancies regardless of mode of delivery.[22,23] In a meta-analysis, a TOL at term was associated with a maternal mortality of 1.9 per 100,000 versus 9.6 per 100,000 for a repeat CD (relative risk [RR], 0.27).[24] Higher rates of maternal mortality were found when including studies that had both preterm and term deliveries; however, the trend of decreased maternal mortality with a TOL persisted.[24]

Uterine rupture
On meta-analysis, the rate of uterine rupture for all women with a history of 1 previous CD is 0.3%, and the rate of uterine rupture is significantly higher for women who

Table 1
Selected outcomes following a trial of labor after cesarean versus a repeat cesarean

Outcome	RR[a]	95% CI
Maternal mortality: all GA	0.33	0.13–0.88
Term	0.27	0.19–0.85
Uterine rupture	20.74	9.77–44.02
Hysterectomy	0.40	0.18–0.92
Transfusion	1.30	1.15–1.47
Maternal fever	0.63	0.43–0.91
Perinatal mortality	1.82	1.24–2.76

Abbreviations: GA, gestational age; RR, relative risk.
[a] RR for a TOLAC compared with repeat CD.
Data from Guise JM, Eden K, Emeis C, et al. Vaginal birth after cesarean: new insights. Evidence report/technology assessment no.191. (Prepared by the Oregon Health & Science University Evidence-based Practice Center under contract no. 290-2007-10057-I). AHRQ Publication No. 10-E003. Rockville (MD): Agency for Healthcare Research and Quality; 2010.

undergo a TOL compared with a repeat CD (0.47% vs 0.026%; *P*<.001).[24] The risk of uterine rupture is higher at term than it is at earlier gestational ages, but most of the high-quality studies on uterine rupture are not stratified by spontaneous versus induced labor, thereby limiting the conclusions that can be made from their results.[24]

Uterine rupture: impact of induction of labor

The risk of uterine rupture with induction of labor (IOL), regardless of induction agent or gestational age, is 1.2%.[24] In the Agency For Healthcare Research And Quality (AHRQ) meta-analysis, IOL was associated with a 0.1% risk difference of uterine rupture at any gestational age, with a greater risk during postterm IOL.[24] Of note, no uterine ruptures were reported during preterm IOL in the included studies.[24] Two recent studies from 2015 examined the risk of uterine rupture secondary to an induced TOLAC versus expectant management.[25,26] In one study of 12,676 women, investigators found no increased risk of rupture with IOL except at gestational ages 39 + 0 to 39 + 6 weeks (1.4% vs 0.5%; aOR, 2.73; 95% CI, 1.22–6.12).[25] In contrast, the second study examined 6033 women from the Consortium on Safe Labor database who attempted TOLAC, and did not find an increased risk of uterine rupture associated with TOL. The investigators reported a uterine rupture rate of 0.2% for the IOL group versus 0.3% for the expectant management group (aOR, 0.72; 95% CI, 0.24–2.17).[26]

The literature regarding the safety of different IOL methods is conflicting. On meta-analysis the uterine rupture rate was 1.1% with oxytocin, 2% with prostaglandin E2, and 6% with misoprostol.[24] Two smaller studies noted no uterine ruptures when mechanical cervical ripening (eg, with a Foley catheter) was used.[24] Based on these results, the 2010 ACOG practice bulletin on VBAC recommended against the use of misoprostol and instead stated, "given the lack of compelling data suggesting increased risk with mechanical dilation and trans-cervical catheters, such interventions may be an option for TOLAC candidates with an unfavorable cervix."[16] At present, there is insufficient evidence to determine the uterine rupture risk when multiple methods of induction are used sequentially.

Other maternal morbidity

Aside from the risk of uterine rupture, studies have examined other possible maternal morbidities associated with a TOL. When considering the risk of hysterectomy secondary to mode of delivery, a prior meta-analysis found that a TOL at any gestational age was associated with a decreased risk for hysterectomy (0.22%) compared with repeat CD (0.43%) for an RR of 0.40 (95% CI, 0.18–0.92)[24]; however, at term there was no significant difference between TOL (0.14%) and a repeat CD (0.16%).[24] This meta-analysis also assessed the risk of postpartum hemorrhage and need for transfusion with each mode of delivery and found that the pooled risk for transfusion was not significantly different between a TOL (0.9%) and a repeat CD (1.2%).[24] When only assessing term pregnancies, a TOL was associated with a slight increased transfusion risk (0.7%) versus a repeat CD (0.5%) for an RR of 1.30 (95% CI, 1.15–1.47).[24]

The risk of maternal infection during a TOLAC versus a repeat CD is difficult to ascertain secondary to the varying criteria for diagnosis used by different studies. The risk for chorioamnionitis was determined to be higher for a TOL, whereas wound infections are more likely following a repeat CD because of the delivery-specific nature of these infections.[24] Postpartum fever was less associated with a TOL (6.5%) versus a repeat CD (7.2%) for an RR of 0.63 (95% CI, 0.43–0.91),[24] but there was a greater risk of postpartum endometritis after a TOL (0.8%–30% risk) versus a repeat CD (risk of 1.2%–18%).[24] Despite these maternal morbidities, at any gestational age, a TOL is associated with a shorter maternal hospital stay (2.55 days) compared with repeat CD (3.92 days),[24] whereas the risk of venous thromboembolism is lower in women with a successful VBAC following a history of a single CD (0.04%) compared with a repeat CD (0.1%).[27]

Impact on future pregnancies

Future childbearing goals are important to consider when counseling patients regarding the risks of a TOL because recent studies have found that 46% of women with 1 child expect to have another child within the next 5 years.[28] In patients who desire future childbearing, mode of delivery in the index pregnancy can significantly affect the risks of future pregnancies including postoperative complications and the incidence of placenta previa as well as placenta accreta spectrum.

Compared with the first cesarean, additional cesareans progressively increase the rates of placenta accreta, unplanned hysterectomy, blood transfusion of more than 4 units, cystotomy, placenta previa, operative time, hospital length of stay, postpartum endometritis, and the need for postoperative ventilation ($P<.001$).[6] The risk of accreta spectrum increases with the number of previous CDs, from 0.24% with no previous CD to 6.7% with 5 or more CDs,[6] and is associated with massive maternal hemorrhage, disseminated intravascular coagulopathy, renal failure, unanticipated surgery, postoperative return to the operating room, maternal death, and preterm delivery.[6,29] The incidence of a placenta previa also increases when a woman has had a history of prior CD (OR, 1.48–3.95).[24] In the presence of a placenta previa the risk of accreta spectrum was 3% if the woman had 1 previous CD, 11% following 2 previous CDs, 40% following 3 previous CDs, and 61% following 4 previous CDs.[6] Placenta previa alone can also be associated with an increased risk of antepartum, intrapartum, and postpartum maternal hemorrhage, hysterectomy, and preterm delivery.[30] It has been projected that, by 2020, the annual incidence of placenta previa, placenta accreta, maternal death, and cesarean hysterectomy will all be significantly increased.[6,31] Despite the low absolute risk of these complications, their devastating nature necessitates careful review when counseling patients regarding the risks and benefits of a TOL.

Neonatal and Infant Outcomes

Perinatal mortality

Perinatal mortality is defined as a fetal demise after 20 weeks' gestational age through the first 7 days of neonatal life. The perinatal mortality for TOL is 1.3 deaths per 1000 deliveries, and 0.5 deaths per 1000 deliveries for women undergoing a repeat CD for an RR of 1.82 (95% CI, 1.24–2.76; P = .041).[24] The risk of perinatal death in the setting of uterine rupture is 6.2% (95% CI, 1.8%–18.8%).[24]

Neonatal morbidity

Investigators have assessed the relationship between a TOLAC and several neonatal outcomes. Hypoxic-ischemic encephalopathy (HIE) is the most serious nonfatal neonatal outcome and can result in permanent neurologic disability. Although there have been prior studies examining the risk of HIE following a TOLAC versus a repeat CD, to date, no study has used the International Cerebral Palsy Task Force definition of HIE[32] when assessing this risk. One study identified cases of HIE using International Classification of Diseases, Ninth Revision (ICD-9) codes in a California administrative database of 41,450 pregnancies and found that the incidence of HIE was higher in both low-risk (0.89% for TOL vs 0.32% for repeat CD) and high-risk (1.29% for TOL vs 0.20% for repeat CD) pregnancies, but the significance of this difference was not assessed.[33] Apgar scores, although not always predictive of HIE, can often be used to identify at-risk infants. When studied, Apgar scores were not consistently different in infants delivered by a TOLAC versus a repeat CD.[34–37]

When studying the risk of birth trauma secondary to mode of delivery, one group of investigators used a broad definition of birth trauma as well as ICD-9 codes (including fetal malpresentation, operative vaginal delivery, and resultant injuries) and found an increased risk associated with TOLAC versus repeat CD (3.7% vs 0.77%) for an OR of 4.2 (95% CI, 1.1–18.2).[38] Aside from birth trauma, neonatal respiratory distress has also been studied and, in a large meta-analysis, the need for bag-and-mask ventilation was found to be significantly higher following a TOL (5.4%; 95% CI, 3.5%–7.6%) than a repeat CD (2.5%; 95% CI, 0.72%–5.0%).[24] In this same analysis, differences in neonatal intubation rates could not be assessed given the heterogeneity of definitions used in eligible studies.[24]

Given the potential increased neonatal risk of a TOLAC, some investigators have hypothesized that this may subsequently result in heightened postpartum neonatal surveillance. In the AHRQ meta-analysis, there was a significant increase in neonatal sepsis work-up following a TOLAC (23%) versus a repeat CD (13%; P = .0008)[39] but no difference in the incidence of culture-positive sepsis.[40,41] In another study, the difference in suspected neonatal sepsis was greater in patients with a labor epidural (30%) versus those without (6%).[40] When assessing the relationship between method of delivery and neonatal admission to the intensive care unit (ICU), most trials found no difference between TOLAC and repeat CD.[24] One moderately sized study reviewed 672 term pregnancies and found no significant difference in neonatal ICU (NICU) admission rates for successful VBAC (3.7%), failed TOL (8.2%), planned repeat CD with labor (8.7%), and planned repeat CD without labor (9.6%; P = .068).[42] In contrast, another recent study found significantly higher NICU admission rates following a TOLAC as opposed to a repeat CD (26% vs 18%; P = .001), but this difference did not persist when assessing NICU admissions of greater than 4 hours' duration (4.2% for TOL vs 4.4% for repeat CD; P = .9).[39]

One of the concerns regarding neonatal outcomes is how the approach to delivery affects breastfeeding initiation. This question was examined in a large study of 31,511 deliveries that included all births between 20 and 42 weeks' gestation in Ohio from 2006 to 2007 in women with 1 prior cesarean delivery. This study determined that, compared with repeat CD, the odds of breastfeeding initiation at 1 to 2 days of life for successful VBAC was an aOR of 1.42 (95% CI, 1.20–1.56) versus an aOR of 1.15 for failed TOL (95% CI, 1.01–1.32).[43]

PREDICTION OF SUCCESSFUL TRIAL OF LABOR

A failed TOLAC is associated with increased maternal and neonatal morbidity and mortality.[24] Thus, it is important to identify predictors of a successful VBAC. Several factors are associated with a successful TOLAC, including a nonreoccurring indication for CD and a TOL following spontaneous labor.[24] A history of a previous vaginal delivery has been the most consistent predictor of VBAC, conferring a 3-fold to 7-fold increased likelihood of success.[24] Similarly, a history of previous VBAC has been shown to increase the likelihood of successful TOL up to 88% to 93%.[44,45] Alternatively, the chance of achieving a VBAC is decreased in the setting of increasing maternal age, African American race, Hispanic ethnicity, obesity, preeclampsia, short-interval pregnancy, and gestational age more than 40 weeks.[24] Infant weight has not been found to affect TOLAC success.[16,24]

Using the factors discussed earlier, 6 different models have been validated for the successful prediction of VBAC.[38–42,46] Three of these models[40,42,46] were then applied to a Northern Irish cohort and their results compared. The models generated by Smith and colleagues[42] and Grobman and colleagues[40] performed well, with area under the curve (AUC) of 0.74 and 0.72 respectively.[47] Using a predicted VBAC threshold of 72%, the sensitivity and specificity for the Grobman and colleagues[40] model was 73% and 57% respectively and for the Smith and colleagues[42] model was 66% and 72% respectively.[40,42] The model proposed by Grobman and colleagues[40] was subsequently used to generate an online calculator capable of estimating a woman's likelihood of successful VBAC (https://mfmu.bsc.gwu.edu/PublicBSC/MFMU/VGBirthCalc/vagbirth.html).

PREDICTION OF UTERINE RUPTURE

Numerous studies have investigated the maternal and fetal factors that influence the risk of uterine rupture. A history of prior vaginal delivery has consistently been found to be protective against uterine rupture (aOR, 0.26–0.62).[48–52] Alternatively, advancing maternal age (>30 years) increases rupture risk, with an aOR of 2.6 (95% CI, 1.1–6.0) for ages 30 to 39 years and 5.8 (95% CI, 1.6–20.3) for age 40 years and older.[51] Interdelivery interval less than 24 months (aOR, 2.05–2.65)[48–50] and a previous single-layer hysterotomy closure (aOR, 3.95–4.33)[48] were both associated with increased likelihood of uterine rupture. Infant birth weight has not been found to influence uterine rupture risk.[48,50]

The impact of previous hysterotomy type on the rate of uterine rupture was examined, and investigators found a 0.75% risk of uterine rupture with a prior low-transverse uterine incision.[52] The highest uterine rupture risk was 2.47% from a prior low-vertical incision followed by 1.59% secondary to a prior classic, T-shaped, or J-shaped hysterotomy. The lowest risk was 0.63% with an unknown prior hysterotomy type. Based on these results, ACOG concluded that "TOLAC is not contraindicated for women with one previous cesarean delivery with an unknown uterine scar type unless there is a high clinical suspicion of a previous classical uterine incision."[16]

Other predictors of uterine rupture have been explored, including the use of sonographic measurements of myometrial thickness before a TOL. One group of investigators found that a lower uterine segment thickness greater than 3.5 mm had a negative predictive value of 99% for uterine rupture but a positive predictive value of 12%.[53] Given the baseline risk of uterine rupture during a TOLAC of 0.47%,[24] the clinical utility of this technique is questionable.

Intrapartum uterine rupture can be difficult to diagnose initially but is most often accompanied by fetal heart tracing abnormalities, specifically fetal bradycardia, which occurs in up to 70% of cases.[15] Other findings can include vaginal bleeding, new onset of maternal pain, abnormal contraction patterns, and loss of fetal station.[15,54] Investigators reviewed obstetric litigations involving TOLAC and found that 80% of claims were avoidable if TOLAC was limited to women who underwent spontaneous labor, not requiring augmentation, and in the absence of signs of fetal compromise (including repetitive variable decelerations).[55] With this conservative approach, it is difficult to determine the number of missed VBAC opportunities for every case of uterine rupture averted.

TRIAL OF LABOR AFTER CESAREAN IN SPECIAL POPULATIONS
History of 2 Previous Cesarean Deliveries

For women with a history of 2 previous CDs, there has been concern regarding the likelihood of a successful VBAC and the potentially increased risk of uterine rupture. One systematic review of 17 studies included 5666 pregnancies, and determined a pooled VBAC success rate of 72%, a uterine rupture rate of 1.1% for TOL versus 0.11% for repeat CD ($P<.001$), and a hysterectomy rate of 0.40% for TOL versus 0.63% for repeat CD ($P = .14$).[56] However, there were insufficient data to analyze neonatal outcomes, including sepsis, HIE, or mortality. Alternatively, a retrospective review of 1082 women with a history of 2 previous CDs found a successful VBAC rate of 75% with no cases of uterine rupture.[57] When 3757 women undergoing a TOL after 1 CD were compared with 134 women undergoing a TOL after 2 CDs there was a significant increase in the rates of uterine rupture (0.8% vs 3.7%; $P = .001$) and failed TOL (25% vs 38%; $P = .001$).[49]

When assessing the risks of a TOL after 2 CDs, it is important to also acknowledge the increased morbidity of a third CD. Two prior studies have retrospectively investigated the risks of a third CD in more than 16,000 pregnancies.[6,57] The rate of uterine rupture was 1.3%,[57] hysterectomy was 0.9%,[6,57] maternal ICU admission was 0.54%[6] to 4.9%,[57] pulmonary embolus was 0.08%,[6] reoperation rate was 0%[54] to 0.25%,[6] and the maternal death rate was 0%[54] and 0.05%.[6] Both studies reported insignificant perinatal morbidity or mortality.[6,57]

In an effort to prevent some of the risks associated with these pregnancies, one study retrospectively applied the VBAC prediction model proposed by Grobman and colleagues to 369 patients with 2 previous cesareans undergoing a TOL.[40,58] The AUC for the Grobman model was 0.74 with similar predicted and actual VBAC success rates,[58] suggesting that this tool may be useful when discussing mode of delivery in this patient population.

Multifetal Gestation

A TOLAC in the setting of multifetal gestation is complicated by many maternal and fetal factors. There is concern that increased uterine distention could augment the risk of uterine rupture.[24] In addition, following a successful VBAC, malpresentation of the second twin could still result in the need for a repeat CD. Of the 3 largest studies evaluating TOLAC in multifetal gestations, 2 used large national databases and ICD-9 codes to identify cases and controls,[59,60] whereas the third used a prospective Maternal Fetal Medicine Units Network cesarean registry cohort.[61] These 3 studies found that the rates of attempted TOLAC were 33%,[59] 39%,[60] and 45%[61] respectively, and the rates of successful VBAC were 76%,[59] 45%,[60] and 65%.[61] In the third study, almost half of the failed TOLAC deliveries occurred following vaginal delivery of the first twin.[61] Another large cohort study found that the rate of uterine rupture was 1.1% during TOLAC, 0.1% during repeat CD, 0.2% with successful VBAC, and 1.4% during failed TOLAC.[59]

When comparing TOLAC in multifetal gestation with singleton gestations, investigators found a significant increase in transfusion risk without increased risks of uterine rupture, bladder/bowel injuries, uterine artery laceration, or postpartum fever.[59] Alternatively, when comparing multifetal TOLAC versus repeat CD there was an increased risk of uterine rupture (RR, 13.7; 95% CI, 4.0–47.0) with no significant differences in the rate of uterine dehiscence, hysterectomy, transfusion, major postpartum infection, postpartum venous thromboembolism, or pelvic hematoma.[60] Alternatively, in the Maternal Fetal Medicine Units Network cesarean registry, investigators found no significant difference in adverse maternal events or perinatal outcomes when comparing multifetal TOLAC versus repeat CD, or when comparing multifetal TOLAC versus singleton TOLAC.[61]

Malpresentation and External Cephalic Version

There are very limited data on the safety of external cephalic version (ECV) in the setting of previous CD.[11] In a retrospective review of 42 pregnancies, investigators found a 72% ECV success rate and a successful VBAC rate of 60%, including failed ECV, with no immediate complications.[62] Based on these results, ACOG recommends that, "external cephalic version is not contraindicated if a woman is at low risk of adverse maternal or neonatal outcomes from [ECV] or TOLAC."[11]

SUMMARY

With the increasing CD rate in the United States, increasing the availability of TOLAC is important to decrease maternal and fetal morbidity associated with repeat CD. In pregnancies complicated by a history of previous CD, both a TOL and a repeat CD are safe options for delivery with overall low absolute rates of adverse maternal or fetal outcomes. Although a repeat CD is associated with increased maternal risks, most of these risks can be anticipated. In comparison, the success of a TOLAC is unpredictable. If a VBAC is achieved, it confers decreased risks to both the mother and the infant, but, if the TOLAC fails, there is a greater risk to both. Because individual women have different risk thresholds, the discussion regarding mode of delivery should begin early in the outpatient prenatal care setting and continue throughout the pregnancy. The discussion surrounding informed consent should incorporate the woman's future childbearing desires, and the woman's specific risk factors and likelihood of success should be documented.

Contemporary data regarding the risks of TOLAC in low-risk and high-risk populations are needed. In addition, prospective studies must be undertaken to determine the safety and efficacy of different induction methods, including mechanical ripening agents versus oxytocin, in addition to the optimal timing of IOL. Barriers to TOLAC availability need to be elucidated and addressed. Providers need to be educated about the risks and benefits of TOLAC, encouraged to use predictive models, and urged to standardize their counseling methods to ensure patient comprehension. Quality metrics are also crucial to determine the number of women attempting TOLAC, VBAC success rates, and incidence of abnormal placentation in order to further educate providers regarding the scope of the issue.

REFERENCES

1. Martin JA, Hamilton BE, Osterman MJK, et al. Births: final data for 2015. Natl Vital Stat Rep 2017;66(1):1.
2. Lydon-Rochelle MT, Cahill AG, Spong CY. Birth after previous cesarean delivery: short-term maternal outcomes. Semin Perinatol 2010;34(4):249–57.

3. Silver RM. Delivery after previous cesarean: long-term maternal outcomes. Semin Perinatol 2010;34(4):258–66.
4. Kolas T, Saugstad OD, Daltveit AK, et al. Planned cesarean versus planned vaginal delivery at term: comparison of newborn infant outcomes. Am J Obstet Gynecol 2006;195(6):1538–43.
5. Geller EJ, Wu JM, Jannelli ML, et al. Neonatal outcomes associated with planned vaginal versus planned primary cesarean delivery. J Perinatol 2010;30(4): 258–64.
6. Silver RM, Landon MB, Rouse DJ, et al. Maternal morbidity associated with multiple repeat cesarean deliveries. Obstet Gynecol 2006;107(6):1226–32.
7. Cragin E. Conservatism in obstetrics. NY Med J 1916;104:1.
8. Schmitz HE, Gajewski CH. Vaginal delivery following cesarean section. Am J Obstet Gynecol 1951;61:1232–42.
9. Cosgrove RA. Management of pregnancy and delivery following cesarean delivery. J Am Med Assoc 1951;145:884–8.
10. National Institutes of Health. Consensus development conference on cesarean childbirth (pub. number 82:2067). Washington, DC: National Institutes of Health; 1981.
11. Gregory KD, Frisman M, Korst L, et al. Trends and patterns of vaginal birth after cesarean availability in the United States. Semin Perinatol 2010;34:237–43.
12. Martin JA, Hamilton BE, Sutton PD, et al. Births: final data for 2004. Natl Vital Stat Rep 2006;55(1):1–101.
13. Martin JA, Hamilton BE, Sutton PD, et al. Births: final data for 2006. Natl Vital Stat Rep 2009;57:1–102.
14. McMahon MJ, Luther ER, Bowes WA, et al. Comparison of a trial of labor with an elective second cesarean section. N Engl J Med 1996;335:689–95.
15. Uddin SF, Simon AE. Rates and success rates of trial of labor after cesarean delivery in the United States, 1990-2009. Matern Child Health J 2013;17:1309–14.
16. American College of Obstetricians and Gynecologists. Practice bulletin 115 vaginal birth after previous cesarean delivery. Washington, DC: ACOG; 2010 (reaffirmed 2015).
17. Barger MK, Dunn JT, Bearman S, et al. A survey of access to trial of labor in California hospitals in 2012. BMC Pregnancy Childbirth 2013;13:83.
18. Leeman LM, Beagle M, Espey E, et al. Diminishing availability of trial of labor after cesarean delivery in New Mexico hospitals. Obstet Gynecol 2013;122:242–7.
19. Bonanno C, Clausing M, Berkowitz R. VBAC: a medicolegal perspective. Clin Perinatol 2011;38:217–25.
20. American College of Obstetrician Gynecologists. ACOG survey on professional liability. Washington, DC: American College of Obstetrician Gynecologists; 2009.
21. Berstein SN, Matalon-Grazi S, Rosenn BM, et al. Trial of labor versus repeat cesarean: are patients making an informed decision? Am J Obstet Gynecol 2012; 207:204.e1-6.
22. Hoyert DL, Hoyert DL. Maternal mortality and related concepts. Vital Health Stat 3 2007;(33):1–13.
23. Kung HC, Hoyert DL, Xu J, et al. Deaths: final data for 2005. Natl Vital Stat Rep 2007;55(19):1–119.
24. Guise J-M, Eden K, Emeis C, et al. Vaginal birth after cesarean: new insights. Evidence report/technology assessment no.191. (Prepared by the Oregon Health & Science University Evidence-based Practice Center under contract no. 290-2007-10057-I). AHRQ Publication No. 10-E003. Rockville (MD): Agency for Healthcare Research and Quality; 2010.

25. Palatnik A, Grobman WA. Induction of labor versus expectant management for women with a prior cesarean delivery. Am J Obstet Gynecol 2015;212:358.e1-6.
26. Lappen JR, Hackney DN, Bailit JL. Outcomes of term induction in trial of labor after cesarean delivery. Obstet Gynecol 2015;126(1):115–23.
27. Landon MB, Hauth JC, Leveno KJ, et al. Maternal and perinatal outcomes associated with a trial of labor after prior cesarean delivery. N Engl J Med 2004; 351(25):2581–9.
28. Daugherty J, Martinez G. Birth expectations of US women aged 15-44. NCHS Data Brief 2016;(260):1–8.
29. Glaze S, Ekwalanga P, Roberts G, et al. Peripartum hysterectomy: 1999-2006. Obstet Gynecol 2008;111:732.
30. Rosenberg T, Pariente G, Sergienko R, et al. Clinical analysis of risk factors and outcome of placenta previa. Arch Gynecol Obstet 2011;284:47.
31. Solheim KN, Esakoff TF, Little SE, et al. The effect of cesarean delivery rates on the future incidence of placenta previa, placenta accreta, and maternal mortality. J Matern Fetal Neonatal Med 2011;24(11):1341–6.
32. Hankin G, Speer M. Defining the pathogenesis and pathophysiology of neonatal encephalopathy and cerebral palsy. Obstet Gynecol 2003;102(3):628–36.
33. Gregory KD, Korst LM, Friedman M, et al. Vaginal birth after cesarean: clinical risk factors associated with adverse outcome. Am J Obstet Gynecol 2008;198(4): 452.e1-10.
34. Fisler RE, Cohen AC, Ringer SA, et al. Neonatal outcome after trial of labor compared with elective repeat cesarean section. Birth 2003;30(2):83–8.
35. Hook B, Kiwi R, Amini SB, et al. Neonatal morbidity after elective repeat cesarean section and trial of labor. Pediatrics 1997;100(3 Pt 1):348–53.
36. Smith GCS, Pell JP, Camerson AD, et al. Risk of perinatal death associated with labor after previous cesarean delivery in uncomplicated term pregnancies. JAMA 2002;287(20):2684–90.
37. Kamath BD, Todd JK, Glazner JE, et al. Neonatal outcomes after elective cesarean delivery. Obstet Gynecol 2009;133(6):1231–8.
38. Hashima JN, Guise J-M. Vaginal birth after cesarean: a prenatal scoring tool. Am J Obstet Gynecol 2007;196(5):e22–3.
39. Flamm BL, Geiger AM. Vaginal birth after cesarean delivery: an admission scoring system. Obstet Gynecol 1997;90(6):907–10.
40. Grobman WA, Lai Y, Landon MB, et al. Development of a nomogram for prediction of vaginal birth after cesarean delivery. Obstet Gynecol 2007;109(4):806–12.
41. Macones GA, Hausman N, Edelstein R, et al. Predicting outcomes of trials of labor in women attempting vaginal birth after cesarean delivery: a comparison of multivariate methods with neural networks. Am J Obstet Gynecol 2001;184(3): 409–13.
42. Smith GCS, White IR, Pell JP. Predicting cesarean section and uterine rupture among women attempting vaginal birth after prior cesarean section. PLoS Med 2005;2(9):e252, 0872-0878.
43. Regan J, Thompson A, DeFranco E. The influence of mode of delivery on breastfeeding initiation in women with a prior cesarean delivery: a population-based study. Breastfeed Med 2013;8(2):181–6.
44. Mercer BM, Gilbert S, Landon MB, et al. Labor outcomes with increasing number of previous prior vaginal births after cesarean delivery. Obstet Gynecol 2008; 111(2 pt 1):285–91.
45. Caughey AB, Shipp TD, Repke JT, et al. Trial of labor after cesarean delivery: the effect of previous vaginal delivery. Am J Obstet Gynecol 1998;179(4):938–41.

46. Troyer LR, Parisi VM. Obstetric parameters affecting success in a trial of labor: designation of a scoring system. Am J Obstet Gynecol 1992;167(4 pt 1): 1099–104.
47. Mone F, Harrity C, Mackie A, et al. Vaginal birth after caesarean section prediction models: a UK comparative observational study. Eur J Obstet Gynecol Reprod Biol 2015;193:136–9.
48. Bujold E, Bujold C, Hamilton EF, et al. The impact of single-layer closure or double-closure on uterine rupture. Am J Obstet Gynecol 2002;186(6):1326–30.
49. Caughey AB, Shipp TD, Repke JT, et al. Rate of uterine rupture during a trial of labor in women with one or two prior cesarean deliveries. Am J Obstet Gynecol 1999;181(4):872–6.
50. Landon MB, Spong CY, Thom E, et al. Risk of uterine rupture with a trial of labor in women with multiple and single prior cesarean delivery. Obstet Gynecol 2006; 108(1):12–20.
51. Shipp TD, Zelop C, Lieberman E. Assessment of the rate of uterine rupture at the first prenatal visit: a preliminary evaluation. J Matern Fetal Neonatal Med 2008; 21(2):129–33.
52. Sprong CY, Landon MB, Gilbert S, et al. Risk of uterine rupture and adverse perinatal outcome at term after cesarean delivery. Obstet Gynecol 2007;110(4): 801–7.
53. Rozenberg P, Goffinet F, Phillippe HJ, et al. Ultrasonographic measurement of lower uterine segment to assess risk of defects of scarred uterus. Lancet 1996; 347(8997):281–4.
54. Grobman WA, Lai Y, Landon MB, et al. Prediction of uterine rupture associated with attempted vaginal birth after cesarean delivery. Am J Obstet Gynecol 2008;199(1):30.e1-5.
55. Clark SL, Belfort MA, Dildy GA, et al. Reducing obstetric litigation through alterations in practice patterns. Obstet Gynecol 2008;112(6):1279–83.
56. Tahseen S, Griffiths M. Vaginal birth after two caesarean sections (VBAC-2) – a systematic review with meta-analysis of success rate and adverse outcomes of VBAC-2 versus VBAC-1 and repeat (third) caesarean sections. BJOG 2010; 117:5–19.
57. Cahill AG, Tuuli M, Odibo AO, et al. Vaginal birth after caesarean for women with three of more prior caesareans: assessing safety and success. BJOG 2010;117: 422–8.
58. Metz TD, Allshouse AA, Faucett AM, et al. Validation of vaginal birth after cesarean delivery prediction model in women with two prior cesareans. Obstet Gynecol 2015;125(4):948–52.
59. Cahill AC, Stamilio DM, Pare E, et al. Vaginal birth after cesarean (VBAC) attempt in twin pregnancies: is it safe? Am J Obstet Gynecol 2005;193:1050–5.
60. Ford AAD, Bateman BT, Simpson LL. Vaginal birth after cesarean delivery in twin gestations: a large, nationwide sample of deliveries. Am J Obstet Gynecol 2006; 195:1138–42.
61. Varner MW, Leindecker S, Sprong CY, et al. The Maternal Fetal Medicine Unit cesarean registry: trial of labor with a twin gestation. Am J Obstet Gynecol 2005; 193:135–40.
62. Sela HY, Fiegenberg T, Ben-Meir A, et al. Safety and efficacy of external cephalic version for women with a previous cesarean delivery. Eur J Obstet Gynecol Reprod Biol 2009;142:111–4.

Quality Improvement and Patient Safety on Labor and Delivery

Bethany Sabol, MD*, Aaron B. Caughey, MD, PhD

KEYWORDS

- Labor and delivery • Quality improvement • Communication • Teamwork
- Maternal outcomes • Neonatal outcomes

KEY POINTS

- Creating a culture of safety and continuous quality improvement should be a priority for all labor and delivery units.
- Key components of patient safety efforts include effective communication, multidisciplinary care and team training, simulation, clinical guidelines, and checklists.
- Implementation of evidence-based quality improvement initiatives endorsed by the American College of Obstetrics and Gynecologists can help to standardize and improve patient care on labor and delivery.

INTRODUCTION

Every component of a health care team shares a common thread, that we are human beings, and despite all of our best efforts, human beings make mistakes. *To Err is Human: Building a Safer Health System,* an Institute of Medicine report, identified that approximately 44,000 Americans die annually from medical errors, making it the eighth leading cause of death in the United States.[1] This number does not take into account near misses or error-related injuries and resultant patient morbidity, nor does it reflect the cost to the health care system and the nation in the form of hospital costs, lost wages, and long-term disability. Perhaps even more important, it fails to capture the loss of trust in the system for both patients and providers.

The obstetric patient population is unique in that the majority of our patients are young and healthy, and childbirth has become a relatively safe event leading to fewer adverse outcomes in this cohort. With that being said, when an adverse event occurs for either mother or child, it can have a catastrophic and lasting effect. A study evaluating adverse events and potential adverse events on labor and delivery confirmed

Department of Obstetrics and Gynecology, Oregon Health and Science University, 3181 SW Sam Jackson Park Road, Portland, OR 97239-3098, USA
* Corresponding author.
E-mail address: sabolb@wustl.edu

Obstet Gynecol Clin N Am 44 (2017) 667–678
http://dx.doi.org/10.1016/j.ogc.2017.08.002
0889-8545/17/© 2017 Elsevier Inc. All rights reserved.

obgyn.theclinics.com

an overall low risk of severe adverse events, but did report that 5% of their patients experienced a quality problem, with 87% of those as a result of a medical error that could have been prevented.[2] These examples highlight the failures of our complex health care system in obstetrics and makes it glaringly obvious that our existing systems fails to build safety into our processes.

Over the last 2 decades, there has been an emphasis on redesigning our health care system to not only eliminate medical errors, but also to create a culture of safety. Within Obstetrics and Gynecology, the American College of Obstetrics and Gynecologists (ACOG) defines a culture of safety as an environment in which all of the types of care providers are empowered to identify errors, near misses, and risky behaviors, and to take part in identifying broader systems issues and engage in active collaboration to improve on and resolve process and system failures.[3]

This article reviews key components that promote a culture of safety and help to move the needle toward the implementation of safer and effective, evidence-based quality care on labor and delivery units. Specifically, it focuses on aspects and examples of how communication, multidisciplinary care, simulation, and the development and implementation of evidence-based, standardized checklists, clinical guidelines, and quality improvement initiatives are moving toward these goals.

COMMUNICATION

Effective communication is the cornerstone of our work. Furthermore, patient perceptions of communication breakdowns can equate to feelings of distrust, dissatisfaction with care, and, in the event of an adverse outcome, medicolegal action.[4] The Joint Commission on Accreditation of Healthcare Organizations (JCAHO) is a not-for-profit organization that focuses on hospital standards and improvement in quality and patient safety. They recommend active involvement in performing root cause analyses for all sentinel events. A root cause analysis is a multidisciplinary systematic exercise designed to identify flaws in a system to prevent errors from happening again. In a review of sentinel events reported to JCAHO, the top listed root cause leading to an infant death or permanent disability was communication issues.[5]

Standardized Terminology

Effective communication needs to start with a common language. In obstetrics, not only is our daily work affected by a lack of common terms, but data collection and meaningful measurement is impossible without standard definitions and the use of these in clinical documentation. In 2011, ACOG and the members of the Women's Health Registry Alliance collaborated to develop standard definitions across the field, called the reVITALize Initiative. These consensus definitions are intended to be incorporated into clinical practice enhancing both clinical communication and allowing for the development of robust national research.[6]

For example, postpartum hemorrhage is a significant cause of maternal morbidity and the most preventable cause of maternal mortality.[7] Historically, postpartum hemorrhage has been defined as an estimated blood loss of more than 500 mL for a vaginal delivery and more than 1000 mL for a cesarean delivery. However, blood loss of more than 500 mL for any mode of delivery, a 10% decrease in hematocrit, a 3 g/dL decrease in hemoglobin, or significant symptoms including lightheadedness, syncope, tachycardia, hypotension, or oliguria, have all also been used.[8] The significant variability in the definition of postpartum hemorrhage has made it difficult to evaluate its true incidence and study interventions to decrease its occurrence. In 2014, ACOG released its reVITALize definition for early postpartum hemorrhage, defining it as a "cumulative blood loss ≥1000 mL or blood loss accompanied by signs/symptoms of hypovolemia within 24 hours following the birth process (includes intrapartum loss)."[9] This definition has been found to be a valid threshold regardless of mode of delivery and accurately predicts a decrease in hemoglobin of more than 3 g/dL and the need for uterotonics.[8] Armed with 49 new, standardized, ACOG-supported definitions, it is imperative that we, as a specialty, incorporate these definitions into practice.

Structured Systems to Enhance Communication

Improved communication on labor and delivery units can be achieved through well-studied, structured tools that are designed to enhance team-based communication. Team huddles, debriefings after sentinel or adverse events, clarification or check-backs, hand-off tools like Situation–Background–Assessment–Recommendation, and conflict resolution using chain of command or 2-challenge rule are all ways of achieving collaboration and improved communication skills on labor and delivery.[10]

A clinical scenario that exemplifies the importance of both a shared, standardized language and structured systems to enhance multidisciplinary team communication is the interpretation of fetal heart rate tracings. Allegations surrounding the interpretation and management of fetal tracing is one of the most cited reasons for malpractice suits and miscommunication between care providers plays a large role in this occurrence. Establishment of nomenclature defined by the National Institute of Child Health and Human Development, training of all care providers who play a role in the interpretation of fetal tracings, and consideration of implementing a protocoled approach to abnormal tracings that incorporate clinical judgment and build in team-based checkins and communication regarding concerns. Consideration of adaptation of protocols and guidelines surrounding a unit's approach to fetal heart rate tracing can help to develop common knowledge structures or "shared mental models," fostering clinical consensus.[11] Furthermore, the development of an electronic fetal monitoring training and certification program for all care providers is another method of identifying knowledge gaps and confirming use of standardized clinical interpretation.[11]

MULTIDISCIPLINARY TEAM TRAINING

A major contributor to adverse events in obstetrics can be traced back to deficiencies in communication and teamwork. In flight training, Crew Resource Management training programs focus on communication and development of shared behaviors to prevent errors and improve safety especially in crisis situations. These programs have proven effective in the aviation world and have been successfully implemented with promising results in other fields, including health care. Training sessions provide clinical teams with improved communication, team building, the ability to recognize emergency situations, decision making, dealing with fatigue, and debriefing and providing feedback.[12]

In obstetrics, these training sessions can be carried out as half-day seminars or multiday courses with a focus on skill development exhibited by highly effective teams, including leadership skills, enhanced communications skills, development of error reduction strategies, and establishing shared vision including modeling of structured communication events such as huddles and debriefings.[4,13] Furthermore, an essential aspect of this team-based learning in obstetrics is that it is multidisciplinary in nature with the incorporation of all aspects of the care team including nurses, obstetricians, midwives, family medicine providers, anesthesiologists, pediatricians, neonatologists, and other staff.

Implementation of this type of multidisciplinary team training in obstetrics is still in its infancy, but the studies evaluating its benefits thus far are promising. One study demonstrated that a team-based training modality in an academic labor and delivery unit resulted in a significant decrease in adverse obstetric outcomes, as well as a 62% decrease in reserved claims resulting from severe adverse events.[12,13] This finding, in combination with literature from other fields of medicine, holds promise that the widespread incorporation of teamwork training will improve patient safety and maternal and neonatal outcomes.[12,14]

SIMULATION

Simulation-based team training is quickly becoming another integral tool for improving patient safety and outcomes in health care. In other specialties, it has been shown to improve teamwork and clinical performance in both simulated and clinical care settings.[15] In obstetrics, rare emergency situations such as a shoulder dystocia, postpartum hemorrhage, eclamptic seizure, and fetal bradycardia can happen at any time and have the potential for possible catastrophic outcomes. Simulation is used to train providers both to technically handle these scenarios and how to effectively communicate through a specific emergency situation.[16] The strength of simulation training is that it allows people to practice together in a safe environment and can identify and mitigate common clinical errors that can occur during an emergency.[17]

The positive effects of multidisciplinary simulation-based team training has been shown in shoulder dystocia simulation with demonstrable improvements in successful deliveries with sustained improvement at the 6- and 12-month follow-up after simulation.[15,18] Furthermore, studies have demonstrated that clinicians who participated in obstetric simulation not only showed significant increases in fund of knowledge, but also improved performance when compared with didactic-based learning strategies.[15] Continued efforts to develop and incorporate simulation-based training into labor and delivery units is an important step in providing improved situational handling of high-risk events, identification of clinical knowledge gaps, and systems issues leading to potential adverse outcomes.

STANDARDIZATION OF CLINICAL PRACTICE

Standardization of processes helps to eliminate variation and has been used successfully to enhance performance and reliability in aviation, the military, and the nuclear energy industry. The use of protocols and checklists in medicine has been shown to decrease medical errors through standardized practice and workflows.[19] In obstetrics, the development of clinical guidelines and standard practice has been challenging given the overall lack of evidence-based practices. It is imperative that physicians and other care providers take an active leadership role in the design, development, and implementation of these protocols and standards. If clinicians do not take the lead as quality becomes increasingly a focus of payers, the government, and private industries, we run the risk of having these guidelines and protocols externally crafted and mandated for us.[19]

The United States has seen an increase in maternal mortality and severe maternal morbidity over the past 5 years, despite overall decreasing rates globally.[20] The most preventable causes have been identified as obstetric hemorrhage, severe hypertension in pregnancy, and peripartum venous thromboembolism.[20] As a response, the National Partnership of Maternal Safety (NPMS) was created as a collaborative national effort to improve maternal safety. This initiative has led to the development of checklists and consensus bundles for management addressing obstetric hemorrhage, severe hypertension in pregnancy, and venous thromboembolism prophylaxis as well as the development of early warning systems in obstetrics. The recommendations of the NPMS bundles are intended to be implemented in every maternity unit. Adaptation to meet the unique specifications of each individual facility is inevitable, but standardization of these implemented bundles within a given institution should be encouraged.[7,20,21]

Checklists

Checklists are informative memory aid tools that ensure completeness and consistency while simultaneously eliminating unnecessary variation that can lead to medical errors. The most well-known example of checklist use in obstetrics is the surgical team pause. This time-out before cesarean delivery and other surgeries taking place on labor and delivery act as a hard stop to ensure that all participating parties agree with the planned procedure and that all concerns have been addressed before proceeding. This check includes ensuring important patient risk factors have been addressed, antibiotics have been given, pneumatic compression devices are on, and the pediatrics team has been called. Another adaptation that has been implemented in some institutions is a checklist at the time of operative vaginal delivery to ensure the appropriateness and readiness for the procedure (fetal position, station, complete dilatation, bladder emptied).[22] The implementation of surgical checklists in medicine have been associated with significant decreases in both surgical complications and mortality[22]; certainly, further implementation and evaluation of their use in obstetrics is imperative.

Clinical Guideline: Obstetric Hemorrhage

As discussed, obstetric hemorrhage is a frequent and significant cause of severe maternal morbidity and mortality. The NPMS has developed a safety bundle organized into 4 domains: readiness, recognition and prevention, response, and reporting and system learning (**Box 1**).[7] It endorses the use of ACOG's revised definition of early postpartum hemorrhage, defined as "cumulative blood loss of $\geq$1,000 mL OR blood loss accompanies by signs and symptoms of hypovolemia within 24 hours following the birth process."[9] The readiness domain is designed to prevent delays that account for a significant proportion of adverse outcomes in obstetric hemorrhages through enhanced preparedness. This domain includes the creation of a hemorrhage cart complete with visual aids and necessary supplies stored in an immediately available location on labor and delivery. It also recommends immediate access to medication while still complying with safe and secure standards. It calls for the creation of a response team in the setting of a severe hemorrhage composed of a maternity provider and a nurse; the team may also include anesthesia, blood bank, interventional radiology, and any other pertinent service and recommends the development of an alert system similar to a code team. Finally, it calls for the development of massive transfusion protocols specific to the unit and regular unit-based simulation and debriefing.[7]

The second domain, recognition and prevention, incorporates screening of every patient to assess their hemorrhage risk, reevaluating their risk throughout labor, and anticipatory planning, when possible, for antepartum patients with significant risk factors (such as Jehovah's Witness or placenta accreta). It is pertinent to remember, however, the need for universal surveillance given that severe postpartum hemorrhage happens in 40% of women without risk factors.[7] Furthermore, accurately assessing cumulative blood loss is essential. The dated estimated blood loss is significantly imprecise, underestimating blood loss in 33% to 50% of cases and acting as a driver

---

Box 1

Obstetric hemorrhage safety bundle from the National Partnership for Maternal Safety, Council on Patient Safety in Women's Health Care

Readiness (every unit)

1. Hemorrhage cart with supplies, checklist, and instruction cards for intrauterine balloons and compression stitches.

2. Immediate access to hemorrhage medications (kit or equivalent).

3. Establish a response team—who to call when help is needed (blood bank, advanced gynecologic surgery, other support and tertiary services).

4. Establish massive and emergency release transfusion protocols (type O negative or uncrossmatched).

5. Unit education on protocols, unit-based drills (with postdrill debriefs).

Recognition and prevention (every patient)

6. Assessment of hemorrhage risk (prenatal, on admission, and at other appropriate times).

7. Measurement of cumulative blood loss (formal, as quantitative as possible).

8. Active management of the third stage of labor (department-wide protocol).

Response (every hemorrhage)

9. Unit-standard, stage-based obstetric hemorrhage emergency management plan with checklists.

10 Support program for patients, families, and staff for all significant hemorrhages.

Reporting and systems learning (every unit)

11. Establish a culture of huddles for high-risk patients and postevent debriefs to identify successes and opportunities.

12. Multidisciplinary review of serious hemorrhages for systems issues.

13. Monitor outcomes and process metrics in perinatal quality improvement committee.

Data from Main EK, Goffman D, Scavone BM, et al. National Partnership for Maternal Safety: consensus bundle on obstetric hemorrhage. Anesth Analg 2015;121(1):142–8.

---

of delayed management of hemorrhage. This bundle calls for improved direct measurement of blood loss using calibrated under-buttocks drapes, and weighing pad/laps as well as active management of the third stage of labor, specifically oxytocin administration, uterine massage, and cord traction. The third domain is response to hemorrhage. This domain describes 2 key interventions that should occur in every hemorrhage. There should be a detailed and standardized management plan in response to every obstetric hemorrhage. Although uterine atony accounts for 70% of obstetric hemorrhages, the evaluation and identification of obstetric hemorrhage etiology is a critical first step. A standardized, stage-based management plan should be developed and implemented in each maternity unit. This should include triggering vital signs and blood loss for each stage, defined roles and responsibilities for each team member, and the creation of a communication plan for activation of the obstetric hemorrhage protocol, similar to a code blue. Each unit needs to adjust these recommendations to fit their individual capabilities, but several successful examples from California, New York, and Florida can serve as roadmaps for successful implementation.[7] This domain also addresses the bystanders of such a significant and traumatic event, the families. Response to a hemorrhage should include the aftermath and establishment of a system that allows for timely discussion, reassurance, and support for patients and their families. The final domain is reporting and systems learning. This step is critical to continuous quality improvement. By establishing a culture of debriefing and huddles, multidisciplinary review of sentinel events, and monitoring of patient outcomes and process metrics, there is a better chance to develop a sustainable process that improves maternal outcomes.

Clinical Guideline: Management of Hypertension

Hypertensive diseases in pregnancy are a major contributor to maternal mortality and severe maternal morbidity and up to 60% of maternal deaths owing to hypertension are potentially preventable.[20,23] Specifically, systolic hypertension is an important predictor of hemorrhagic stroke and cerebral infarction.[20] The timely identification and treatment of systolic and diastolic blood pressures to prevent stroke and other major morbidities is crucial, and the implementation of standardized order sets and management protocols has resulted in the reduction of severe maternal morbidity and mortality.[20,24] The Severe Hypertension in Pregnancy Working Group of ACOG has developed guidelines for the management of acute-onset severe hypertension in pregnancy and the postpartum period.[24] They recommend that women with acute-onset severe systolic or diastolic hypertension receive urgent antihypertensive therapy (as soon as possible—within 30–60 minutes) with either intravenous labetalol or hydralazine, or oral immediate release nifedipine after confirmed severe hypertension defined as a persistent blood pressure greater than 160/110 mm Hg for 15 minutes or longer. They encourage the development of standardized protocols to measure blood pressure in pregnancy to ensure accuracy (an example of this is the California Maternal Quality Care Collaborative Toolkit for standardized BP measurement). ACOG Committee Opinion 692 provides sample order sets for treatment of severe hypertension with each first-line agent.[24] Finally, they recommend that in the setting of resistant severe hypertension an emergent consultation with anesthesia, maternal–fetal medicine, or critical care subspecialist occur to discuss second-line intervention.

Clinical Guideline: Prevention of Thromboembolism

Venous thromboembolism is a significant cause of maternal morbidity and mortality and is potentially preventable is appropriate risk factor-based prophylaxis. The NPMS in 2016 released a consensus bundle on venous thromboembolism. The bundle is divided into the 4 following domains (**Box 2**).[21] (1) *Readiness* is the establishment of risk throughout pregnancy, specifically during the first prenatal visit, during antepartum admissions, immediately postpartum, and upon discharge home after birth using validated tools modified for obstetric patients (Caprini System or Padua System, modifications online at http://links.lww.com/AOG/A834).[21] (2) *Recognition* expects that, through routine screening, high-risk patients will be identified and be intervened upon accordingly. (3) *Response* outlines the NPMS recommendations for at-risk patient prophylaxis based on available evidence, guidelines from ACOG, the Royal College of Obstetricians and Gynecologists, and the American College of Chest Physicians. **Table 1** presents the current recommendations for thromboprophylaxis. In the setting of cesarean birth, mechanical thromboprophylaxis with pneumatic compression devices should be used for everyone while in bed until hospital discharge and the NPMA acknowledges that using the Royal College of Obstetricians and Gynecologists and Caprini scoring systems identify most women undergoing cesarean as high risk and allows for hospitals to choose a strategy in which all women undergoing cesarean receive postoperative low-molecular-weight heparin. (4) *Reporting and systems learning* calls for individual hospitals to create and implement methods of

---

Box 2
Venous thromboembolism prevention maternal safety bundle

Readiness

Every unit
• Use a standardized thromboembolism risk assessment tool during:
  ○ Outpatient prenatal care,
  ○ Antepartum hospitalization,
  ○ Hospitalization after cesarean or vaginal birth, and
  ○ Postpartum period (up to 6 weeks after birth).

Recognition and prevention

Every patient
• Apply standardized tool to all patients to assess venous thromboembolism risk at time points designated under Readiness.
• Apply standardized tool to identify appropriate patients for thromboprophylaxis.
• Provide patient education.
• Provide all health care providers education regarding risk assessment tools and recommended thromboprophylaxis.

Response

Every unit
• Use standardized recommendations for mechanical thromboprophylaxis.
• Use standardized recommendations for dosing of prophylactic and therapeutic pharmacologic anticoagulation.
• Use standardized recommendations for appropriate timing of pharmacologic prophylaxis with neuraxial anesthesia.

Reporting and systems learning

Every unit
• Review all thromboembolism events for systems issues and compliance with protocols.
• Monitor process metrics and outcomes in a standardized fashion.
• Assess for complications of pharmacologic thromboprophylaxis.

Standardization of health care processes and reduced variation has been shown to improve outcomes and quality of care. The Council on Patient Safety in Women's Health Care disseminates patient safety bundles to help facilitate the standardization process. This bundle reflects emerging clinical, scientific, and patient safety advances as of the date issued and is subject to change. The information should not be construed as dictating an exclusive course of treatment or procedure to be followed. Although the components of a particular bundle may be adapted to local resources, standardization within an institution is strongly encouraged.

Data from D'Alton ME, Friedman AM, Smiley RM, et al. National Partnership for Maternal Safety: consensus bundle on venous thromboembolism. Obstet Gynecol 2016;128(4):688–98.

---

surveillance including determination of underlying prevalence of risk factors for venous thromboembolism to help tailor venous thromboembolism prophylaxis policies based on the population. After implementation, monitoring compliance with risk assessment and appropriate prophylaxis practices as well as review of all cases of obstetric related thromboembolism, monitoring of adverse outcomes with pharmacologic prophylaxis.[21]

Quality Improvement Initiative: The Maternal Early Warning System

The majority of clinical emergencies in obstetrics are preceded by early indicators that hint toward potential instability and clinical decline. Trigger tools are designed to as an aid to help clinicians identify and intervene in a timely manner. The Maternal Early

Table 1
NPMS recommendations for thromboprophylaxis

Antepartum Outpatient Prophylaxis	
Treatment dose LMWH or UFH	Multiple prior VTE episodes Prior VTE with high-risk thrombophilia[a] Prior VTE with acquired thrombophilia[c]
Prophylactic dose LMWH or UFH	Idiopathic prior VTE Prior VTE with pregnancy or oral contraceptives Prior VTE with low-risk thrombophilia[b] High-risk thrombophilia[a]
No treatment	Low-risk thrombophilia Prior provoked VTE Low-risk thrombophilia[b] and family history of VTE
Antepartum inpatient prophylaxis	
Prophylactic dose of LMWH or UFH	Antepartum patients hospitalized for at least 72 h who are not at high risk of bleeding or imminent childbirth
Vaginal birth	
Postpartum prophylactic dose of LMWH or UFH (plus intrapartum pneumatic compression)	History of VTE or thrombophilia High risk (based on RCOG criteria or Padua score $\geq$ 4) may be considered
Cesarean birth	
Prophylactic dose of LMWH or UFH	Women with risk factors
Extended postpartum thromboprophylaxis	
Treatment dose of LMWH or UFH for 6 wk postpartum	Multiple prior VTE episodes Prior VTE with high-risk thrombophilia[a] Prior VTE with acquired thrombophilia[c]
Prophylactic dose of LMWH or UFH for 6 wk postpartum	Idiopathic prior VTE Prior VTE with pregnancy or oral contraceptives Prior VTE with low-risk thrombophilia[b] High-risk thrombophilia (including acquired) Family history of VTE with high-risk thrombophilia[a] Prior provoked VTE Low-risk thrombophilia[b] and family history of VTE
No treatment	Low-risk thrombophilia[b]

Abbreviations: LMWH, low-molecular-weight heparin; NPMS, National Partnership of Maternal Safety; RCOG, Royal College of Obstetricians and Gynecologists Royal College of Obstetricians and Gynecologists; UFH, unfractionated heparin; VTE, venous thromboembolism.

[a] High-risk thrombophilias: factor V Leiden homozygosity, prothrombin gene mutation homozygosity, factor V Leiden, prothrombin gene mutation compound heterozygosity, and antithrombin III deficiency.

[b] Low-risk thrombophilias: factor V Leiden or prothrombin gene mutation heterozygosity and protein C or S deficiency.

[c] Acquired thrombophilia: antiphospholipid antibody syndrome.

Data from D'Alton ME, Friedman AM, Smiley RM, et al. National Partnership for Maternal Safety: consensus bundle on venous thromboembolism. Obstet Gynecol 2016;128(4):688–98.

Warning Criteria is an adaptation of the Modified Early Obstetric Warning System originally developed in the United Kingdom.[17] While highlighting a potentially compromised patient, the Maternal Early Warning Criteria simultaneously mobilizes a corrective action plan in hopes of preventing further escalation. The Maternal Early

Table 2	
Maternal early warning criteria	
Parameter	**Value**
Systolic BP (mm Hg)	<90 or >160
Diastolic BP (mm Hg)	>100
Heart rate (beats/min)	<50 or >120
Respiratory rate (breaths/min)	<10 or >30
Oxygen saturation on room air, at sea level, %	<95
Oliguria, mL/h for ≥2 h	<35
Maternal agitation, confusion, or unresponsiveness; Patient with preeclampsia reporting a nonremitting headache or shortness of breath	

Early warning system proposed by National Partnership for Maternal Safety.
Abbreviation: BP, blood pressure.
From Mhyre JM, D'Oria R, Hameed AB, et al. The maternal early warning criteria: a proposal from the National Partnership for Maternal Safety. Obstet Gynecol 2014;124(4):784; with permission.

Warning Criteria is an example of a trigger tool that successfully facilitates timely response to acute maternal illness (**Table 2**).[22] It is meant to act as a bedside assessment tool that is incorporated like a vital sign into the electronic medical record. Any one abnormal value is meant to trigger physician assessment. In other medical literature, the evidence supporting trigger tools and early warning systems to identify patients needing more acute care is robust. Validation of these tools in obstetrics is still ongoing but implementation of the Maternal Early Warning Criteria has already been associated with improvement in maternal mortality, maternal admissions to the intensive care unit, and rates of maternal bacteremia.[22,25]

SUMMARY

All of these components have significant overlapping and recurring themes centered on communication, preparation, standardization, and teamwork. Together, these components make labor and delivery units a safer place for moms and babies. A Boston-area hospital demonstrated how implementation of these components can lead to improved patient safety and quality reflected by decreased reserve claims. From 2004 to 2009, they revised their provider call schedule limiting the ability of on-call physicians from having clinical responsibilities on their postcall days, initiating an obstetric drill workshop, implementing a collaborative care committee, launching a standardized electronic fetal heart rate monitoring course, creating a dedicated obstetric quality assessment and improvement committee, and requiring cultural competency and teams training. Through this 5-year period they saw their number of reserved claims per delivery decrease at a rate of 20% per policy year. This was interpreted as an overall marker of improved patient safety and quality care.[4]

As obstetricians, we need to be committed to the process of continual quality improvement and need to be leaders in creating a culture of patient safety throughout the environment in which we work. It is impossible to improve on a problem that we do not acknowledge, identify, or measure. Continued work toward the development and validation of evidence-based quality indicators is needed as well as improved systems to detect and review adverse events. Given the overall rarity of severe adverse events it is imperative to design a system that also identifies near misses and quality issues potentiating harm.[2] Finally, we need to look toward the future. Developing and integrating a quality improvement curriculum starting in undergraduate medical education is vital to training all new physicians to think and work with the mindset of quality and patient safety.

REFERENCES

1. Kohn LT, Corrigan J, Donaldson MS. To err is human: building a safer health system. Washington, DC: National Academy Press; 2000.
2. Forster AJ, Fung I, Caughey S, et al. Adverse events detected by clinical surveillance on an obstetric service. Obstet Gynecol 2006;108(5):1073–83.
3. American College of Obstetricians and Gynecologists Committee on Patient Safety and Quality Improvement. ACOG committee opinion no. 447: patient safety in obstetrics and gynecology. Obstet Gynecol 2009;114(6):1424–7.
4. Iverson RE Jr, Heffner LJ. Patient safety series: obstetric safety improvement and its reflection in reserved claims. Am J Obstet Gynecol 2011;205(5):398–401.
5. Grunebaum A. Error reduction and quality assurance in obstetrics. Clin Perinatol 2007;34(3):489–502.
6. Menard MK, Main EK, Currigan SM. Executive summary of the reVITALize initiative: standardizing obstetric data definitions. Obstet Gynecol 2014;124(1):150–3.
7. Main EK, Goffman D, Scavone BM, et al. National partnership for maternal safety: consensus bundle on obstetric hemorrhage. Obstet Gynecol 2015;126(1): 155–62.
8. Hamm RF, Wang EY, Bastek JA, et al. Assessing reVITALize: should the definition of postpartum hemorrhage differ by mode of delivery? Am J Perinatol 2017;34(5): 503–7.
9. ACOG: The American Congress of Obstetricians and Gynecologists. reVITALize. Available at: http://www.acog.org/About-ACOG/ACOG-Departments/Patient-Safety-and-Quality-Improvement/reVITALize. Accessed March 22, 2017.
10. Pettker CM, Grobman WA. Obstetric safety and quality. Obstet Gynecol 2015; 126(1):196–206.
11. Pettker CM. Standardization of intrapartum management and impact on adverse outcomes. Clin Obstet Gynecol 2011;54(1):8–15.
12. Merien AE, van de Ven J, Mol BW, et al. Multidisciplinary team training in a simulation setting for acute obstetric emergencies: a systematic review. Obstet Gynecol 2010;115(5):1021–31.
13. Pratt SD, Mann S, Salisbury M, et al. John M. Eisenberg Patient Safety and Quality Awards. Impact of CRM-based training on obstetric outcomes and clinicians' patient safety attitudes. Jt Comm J Qual Patient Saf 2007;33(12):720–5.
14. Grogan EL, Stiles RA, France DJ, et al. The impact of aviation-based teamwork training on the attitudes of health-care professionals. J Am Coll Surg 2004; 199(6):843–8.
15. Daniels K, Auguste T. Moving forward in patient safety: multidisciplinary team training. Semin Perinatol 2013;37(3):146–50.
16. Gardner R, Raemer DB. Simulation in obstetrics and gynecology. Obstet Gynecol Clin North Am 2008;35(1):97–127, ix.
17. American College of Obstetricians and Gynecologists Committee on Patient Safety and Quality Improvement. Committee opinion no. 590: preparing for clinical emergencies in obstetrics and gynecology. Obstet Gynecol 2014;123(3): 722–5.
18. Crofts JF, Bartlett C, Ellis D, et al. Training for shoulder dystocia: a trial of simulation using low-fidelity and high-fidelity mannequins. Obstet Gynecol 2006;108(6): 1477–85.

19. Committee on Patient Safety and Quality Improvement. Committee opinion no. 629: clinical guidelines and standardization of practice to improve outcomes. Obstet Gynecol 2015;125(4):1027–9.

20. D'Alton ME, Main EK, Menard MK, et al. The national partnership for maternal safety. Obstet Gynecol 2014;123(5):973–7.

21. D'Alton ME, Friedman AM, Smiley RM, et al. National partnership for maternal safety: consensus bundle on venous thromboembolism. Obstet Gynecol 2016; 128(4):688–98.

22. Arora KS, Shields LE, Grobman WA, et al. Triggers, bundles, protocols, and checklists–what every maternal care provider needs to know. Am J Obstet Gynecol 2016;214(4):444–51.

23. Shields LE, Wiesner S, Klein C, et al. Early standardized treatment of critical blood pressure elevations is associated with a reduction in eclampsia and severe maternal morbidity. Am J Obstet Gynecol 2017;216(4):415.e1-5.

24. Committee on Obstetric Practice. Committee opinion no. 692: emergent therapy for acute-onset, severe hypertension during pregnancy and the postpartum period. Obstet Gynecol 2017;129(4):e90–5.

25. Shields LE, Wiesner S, Klein C, et al. Use of maternal early warning trigger tool reduces maternal morbidity. Am J Obstet Gynecol 2016;214(4):527.e1-6.

Moving?

Make sure your subscription moves with you!

To notify us of your new address, find your **Clinics Account Number** (located on your mailing label above your name), and contact customer service at:

Email: journalscustomerservice-usa@elsevier.com

800-654-2452 (subscribers in the U.S. & Canada)
314-447-8871 (subscribers outside of the U.S. & Canada)

Fax number: 314-447-8029

Elsevier Health Sciences Division
Subscription Customer Service
3251 Riverport Lane
Maryland Heights, MO 63043

*To ensure uninterrupted delivery of your subscription,
please notify us at least 4 weeks in advance of move.

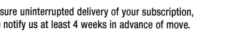

Printed and bound by CPI Group (UK) Ltd, Croydon, CR0 4YY

03/10/2024

01040391-0014